Qi Gong

LEARNING THE WAY

by

Simon Bastian

**GREEN
MAGIC**

Qi Gong - Learning the Way © 2013 by Simon Bastian.

All rights reserved. No part of this book may be used or reproduced in any form without written permission from the author, except in the case of quotations in articles and reviews

Green Magic
5 Stathe Cottages
Stathe
Somerset
TA7 0JL
England

www.greenmagicpublishing.com
email: info@greenmagicpublishing.com

Cover photo by Lynn Bastian

Typeset by Green Man Books, Dorchester
www.greenmanbooks.co.uk

ISBN 978 0 9566197 1 6

GREEN MAGIC

ACKNOWLEDEGMENTS

Again, many thanks and much love to Lynn for support and inspiration; the multi-talented creative genius behind The Wild Hunt (www.thewildhunt.moonfruit.com) and Herotica Art (www.heroticaart.moonfruit.com)

Love and best wishes to Bethan, Eleri, Rose and Ron, Sue and Dex, Pam, Christopher, Lezah and Karl, John and Alison, Hazel, Ian and Jo, Tony and Karen, and Shirley, and to all my family and friends.

My respect and gratitude to Tai Chi and Qi Gong Master John Barber for teaching me the Prenatal Energy exercises among other forms, and to my many other teachers. Thanks also to my students over the years.

The 'Qi Gong' chapter was originally published in abridged form in 'Four Winds' magazine, and part of the chapter 'The Gate of Gifts' appeared as 'Tao and the Western Esoteric Tradition' in 'Conjure', the online magazine. Both magazines were edited and produced by Ellen May Long.

Both Ellen and Martin Potts (www.candocomputing.co.uk) provided much needed assistance in formatting.

The concept of the 'Time, Space and Event Mudra' in 'The Single Palm Change' came from memories of my father reading (as a demonstration of properties in physics, it was invented by the engineer John Ambrose Fleming).

Thanks to Sue Render of Labyrinth Books for publication advice, to my publisher Peter Gotto for expert guidance and advice, and to the team at Green Magic publishing. Fiona Brogan very kindly provided the photography (www.timelessartportraits.co.uk).

Robert Poyton, the country's leading instructor in Systema (and also a great Tai Chi teacher) provided my introduction to this form of martial art.

Most of my knowledge of Dim Mak and the application of the reptilian brain came from the late Erle Montaigue, founder of the World Taiji Boxing Association.

My thanks to Peter Carroll for formative correspondence on Chaos Magic in the early '80s.

The lovely people at Hadean Press, Dis Albion and Erzebet Carr, who published my booklet 'The Glastonbury I Ching', which is also available as a set including trigram discs through The Wild Hunt. Dis also tidied up my Glass Isle Qi Gong logo (as shown on the title page here, consisting of the trigrams, eight pointed star and an early version of the Yin/Yang symbol).

Regards to Jack and Jamie of St Martha's Botanica, who provide a wealth of knowledge in all things esoteric (www.theoccultconsultancy.com).

Finally, in loving memory of my parents, Joseph Douglas and Enid May Bastian.

GLASS ISLE QI GONG

For details of classes and workshops with Simon, email sbglassisleqg@gmail.com or message Glass Isle Qi Gong on Facebook.

CONTENTS

Foreword   vi

The Chinese Language   viii

1. A Brief History of the Middle Kingdom   1
2. The Gate of Gifts: Aspects of Esotericism   5
3. Qi Gong   23
4. The Health Classic   29
5. Breathing   33
6. Sitting   37
7. Standing   41
8. The Meridian Energy Model   47
9. Occult Anatomy   49
10. The 8 Trigrams, 5 Elements and Qi Peak Flow   51
11. The Yuan Qi Exercises   57

12. Walking	83
13. Circle Walking	87
14. The Single Palm Change	93
15. Buddhist Walking	103
16. Geomythic Energy	107
17. Mapping the Many Worlds	111
18. Qabalistic Silk Reeling	115
19. The Internal Martial Arts	125
20. Teaching and Therapy	133
21. Effects and Guidelines	137
22. Stress	139
23. Conclusion - The Te: Morality in an Amoral Universe	143

APPENDICES:

Glossary	146
Personalities	147
A List of the Chinese Dynasties	148
Bibliography	149

FOREWORD

Jung, in his commentary on 'The Secret of the Golden Flower' (a Taoist alchemical work that was translated by Richard Wilhelm), addresses the problem of the Western mindset trying to accommodate Chinese thought. He likened it to the student in Faust who gets carried away by Eastern esoteric practices.

Popular interpretations of Taoism tend toward its apparent vagueness or mysticism, or as a purported adjunct to quantum physics. Actually, magical practice is still a vital part of the Taoist worldview, alongside ceremony and pure philosophical contemplation.

The aims of this book have been both practical and theoretical; to present traditional, lineage Taoist Qi Gong exercises, and to interpret Tao as I understand it, in the light of a Western cultural sensibility. To this end comparisons will be made with what is known as our 'secret history' or esoteric tradition. I hope to provide an insight into how these seemingly diverse lines of thought are not mutually exclusive, by recognizing that the search for optimum means of developing and unfolding human potential naturally arrive at similar methodology, despite dissimilar historical and social backgrounds. The teaching of wisdom has often quite clearly required secrecy due to religious persecution and other reasons. Occultism simply means the study of that which is hidden, as in the astronomical term occultation, and is concerned with the deciphering and revealing of the hidden nature of things, what Schopenhauer interpreted as Will. Each act of Will, performed with complete consciousness, is in some way a magical act. This accords with Taoism's ideal of seeing the sacred within everyday life

With the Taoist practices Prenatal Energy, the original spark of life, is a continuing active force in every individual's existence, and one which can be engaged to enhance our lives. Other traditions also treat of the same principle. The physician William Sutherland, who created Cranial Osteopathy, believed there was a form of corrective energy in his patients, a matrix of original intention that could be accessed to improve health and related to the embryological forces that directed physiological processes.

The great wisdom of the Taoists was formulated in their energetic practices, designed to align the personal with the transpersonal. The Yuan Qi or Primordial Energy exercises described here, along with other Taoist forms of Qi Gong, are just one.

Simon Bastian

Glastonbury 2013

THE CHINESE LANGUAGE

The official, national language is Mandarin Chinese, although there are many dialects, such as Cantonese, that are spoken by millions.

Spoken Chinese is tonal, which means there can be four pronunciations with four different meanings for each word. The composition of the written language is in ideograms, which unlike single alphabetical characters can represent whole concepts and phrases.

There are different systems of transliterating these ideograms into English, including the Wade-Giles, Pinyin and Yale University systems. Qi Gong in Pinyin translates as Chi Kung in the Wade-Giles method. The pronunciation is actually closer to Chee Gung.

Obviously, difficulties arise in interpreting what are in any case abstruse philosophical terms. I have not followed a consistent form of translation, as some terms are more familiar in one system than another. My somewhat idiosyncratic use of the systems is based on this admittedly arbitrary rule of familiarity.

For instance, Tai Chi (Taiji in Pinyin) and Tao (Dao), which incidentally is pronounced 'Dow', are still more recognizable to most people in the Wade-Giles form, whereas the Pinyin spelling of Beijing has now taken over from the old style Peking.

Whatever system is used, English words are just approximations for the spoken ideograms. What really matters is relating the meaning.

Allowing for this academic fault line, I trust the sense of the terms will therefore be adequately conveyed.

QI GONG - LEARNING THE WAY

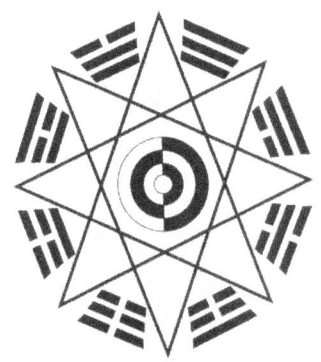

1. A BRIEF HISTORY OF THE MIDDLE KINGDOM

China is quite possibly the oldest continuous civilization in the world. The name for the country could be derived from Qin (pronounced Chin), which comes from the dynasty established by Qin Shi Huang in 221 BC, the first united state. Alternatively its origination may be a Sanskrit word.

Traditionally known as the Middle Kingdom, because it was thought to be the centre of civilization, China's insularity could be considered a consequence of natural geographic position, being bounded by the Tibetan plateau and Gobi desert, but also as a reticence towards contact with outside cultures.

The royal family was founded by Huang Ti, the Yellow Emperor (c.2658-2599 BC), author of the Neijing Suwen, the classic of internal medicine. The establishment of a silk trade route meant Indian Buddhism began to flourish from around the first and second centuries AD, but the country has still maintained a remarkable homogeneity for its immense size, and despite regional ethnic and linguistic differences.

Reflecting upon the agrarian nature of the early culture, it can be understood that ideas such as the balance of Yin and Yang grew out of a deep involvement with the natural world rather than as mere intellectual musing. Divination also held a vital importance, which is understandable in a climate of survivalism, where the safest course of action needed to be established. The I Ching and other arts thus took a primary role in attempting to alleviate fears and aid decision.

With a shifting consciousness of ordering one's own world, the concept of a Supreme Being was replaced by a more impersonal construct, the Way of an implicate reality. Deities were still worshipped but human status had altered.

The authoritarian centralizing effect of the unification of the country led to an hierarchical bureaucracy, and many of the great philosophers were educated and held posts within this structure. The Legalists later placed power within the person of the Emperor during the Chin period, and at this time the Great Wall was built. It was an oppressive regime in which all books were burnt except those that dealt with medical, divinatory and technological subjects. Thankfully the Nei Jing and I Ching were therefore saved.

The more enlightened Han Dynasty that followed allowed scholars to revitalize classic texts and expound upon such matters as the Five Element Theory and Yin/Yang harmony.

During the Tang (618-907) and Song (960-1279) Dynasties, philosophy, art and technology flourished. There was another Golden Age with the Ming Dynasty (1368-1644). However, European Imperialism had a disastrous effect on the nation, British opium in particular contributing to the country's decline. The last Emperor was Puyi, the final member of the Manchu Qing Dynasty, who ruled from 1908 to 1912, then for 12 days in 1917.

Sun Yat-sen founded the Republic of China in 1912, which today governs Taiwan, separated politically from mainland China. The People's Republic of China was proclaimed in 1949.

Buddhism is the most popular form of religion in China, with Taoism second, although the term 'religion' is questioned by some academics, who would prefer to reference them as 'belief systems'. Western religions such as Christianity were introduced during the 18th and 19th centuries with the advent of imperialist ambition. The Communist Party government is officially atheist, and during the Cultural Revolution many places of worship were either converted into secular buildings or destroyed. There was a change of heart in the 1980s with a program to rebuild Buddhist and Taoist temples as examples of Chinese heritage.

Confucianism provides the social, moral background as a value system, and the honouring of ancestors is important. There are as well branches of folk religion, shamanism, cults and ethnic traditions.

Taoism was established as a religion in the time of the Han Dynasty. The T'ai-p'ing Ching (Book of Peace and Balance) was the first appearance of a Taoist religious scripture, equivalent to the Bible, the Tao Te Ching being regarded in contrast as a philosophical work. Around that time Lao Tzu began to be considered a deity, with temples and shrines dedicated to him. Characters such as Chang Tao-ling and K'ou Ch'ien-chih established different branches of religious Taoism.

Magical Taoism is the most ancient form, invoking and accessing the power of differentiated aspects of the Tao as embodied by deities, and working with the elements. The Fang-shih were magicians who could be consulted to provide talismans for improving conditions, such as better health or ensuring crops did not fail. Performance of rituals is an important part of Ceremonial or Devotional Taoism, and there is the more personal Tao of self-cultivation. All these different types were not necessarily incompatible with one another. The general reading of Taoism as being split between philosophical and religious interpretations is not completely true. Shamanic culture was always very influential.

Taoism divided into two main sects after the Yuan Dynasty, the Quanzhen or Complete Reality school, practising Neidan (internal alchemy), and Zhengyi Dao or the Way of Complete Orthodoxy that evolved from the Tianshi Dao, Way of the Celestial Masters.

Lao Tzu (Old Teacher), the popular name for Li Erh, is considered to be the founder of Taoism due to traditionally being regarded as the author of the Tao Te Ching, the Classic of the Way and its Virtue. He was born around 600 BC, although his actual existence is disputed by some authorities. Others claim he was a contemporary of Confucius, and worked as an archivist for the Royal Court. The legend has it that, as he grew tired of life in the city, he was leaving to become a hermit when he was recognized and stopped at the gate by a sentry, who asked for a testament of his knowledge. Whereupon Lao Tzu wrote the Tao Te Ching, then left never to be seen again.

The book describes the Tao as the root of all existence, and advises seeking the state of wu wei, a complex concept of spontaneous action arising from not forcing action, in order to become attuned to it. The Tao Te Ching took its present form around the 3rd century BC, and despite some contention over the matter of authorship, does read cohesively.

Chuang Tzu is another of the great Taoist figures whose life is shrouded in mystery. He is placed in the 4th century BC, and his work is usually known by his name, just as the Tao Te Ching is sometimes called the Lao Tzu.

Chuang Tzu explored and expanded Lao Tzu's teachings. He is very humane and humorous. While his exposition of a relativistic, all embracing transcendentalism has been criticized on the grounds of moral permissiveness, his influence on the concept of self-development is undeniable. Zen Buddhism was founded on his writings.

The Lieh Tzu has controversial sources. As a personality, it is conjectured that he may have been a creation of Chuang Tzu's to express his ideas in a different manner.

Confucius, a Latinization of Kongfutze, lived from 551 to 497 BC. He was a humanist who believed in rationalism and benevolence, and his views influenced Chinese society's ideals of morality and order.

2. THE GATE OF GIFTS: ASPECTS OF ESOTERICISM

I. THE TAO AND CHAOS

There's a line from a Chinese poet; 'Those who know keep silence'.

The problem with writing about Taoism is that, essentially, it's an indefinable subject. The words at the beginning of the 'Tao Te Ching', Lao Tzu's principal text, are, after all, 'The Tao that can be named is not the true Tao'. And even that short sentence has been subject to centuries of speculation and endless variations in interpretation. So I will now proceed to offer several words on a wordless topic.

The ideogram for 'Tao' is composed of the elements for 'Head' and 'Going', which can be interpreted as our intention to travel along the Path, or as leaving the Head Orientation behind and seeking a more holistic quality in life.

The restless urge to define, the inability to simply go with the intangible and vague, are part of the incisive and rational qualities of Western intellectual rigour. Rigour to the point of rigor mortis, it might be said, because evaluation through the logistics of nomenclature, trying to tie every part and parcel of the world down in a neat pigeon hole, avoids that Dweller on the Threshold, direct experience.

When we 'see into the life of things', as Wordsworth put it, it can be a little scary. The Tao is not 'human hearted'; to it, we are as straw dogs. Theologians have attempted to interpret God and Tao as one and the same, but they're not. You do not deify the Tao or call on it for help in time of need, but rather unite with it through meditation and the cultivation of one's self in order to realise the inner workings of reality. Though the Tao of the Tao Te Ching is benevolent, it was later, to Chuang Tzu for example, seen as having a neutral quality. Chuang Tzu said 'Tao abides only in the emptiness'. There did arise household gods and deified aspects in the religious rather than philosophical manifestation, but these are incidental to the fundamental conception.

Pointedly enough, it could be because the Tao lacks 'human' attributions such as Jealousy and Love that religious warfare has seldom been waged in its name (an isolated exception was the persecution and killing of all Buddhists in Northern China during the 4th to 5th Centuries AD, when Taoism was made the state religion). It would seem an outcome of the anthropomorphizing of the Divine is conflict.

There were Taoist sects that became involved in struggles against the state, but they had political motivations, such as support for the downtrodden peasants.

This inhuman quality of Tao does not present a nihilistic slant on existence though. On the contrary, whereas certain schools of thought look upon life and the world as illusory, Taoism is rooted in the physical. Self realisation through daily experience is one core ideal.

And Taoism does not override other beliefs. There are Taoist practitioners who are at the same time devout Christians, Buddhists and believers in other faiths. It is an inclusive path. The Chinese have had a wonderfully utilitarian and pragmatic approach to the different schools of religion. Hence they could mix and match praying to Buddhist and/or Taoist deities whilst following the Confucian moral code, quite a refreshing contrast to certain dogmatic religions which have tended to exterminate deviants. Buddha and Lao Tzu were often conflated as one being. There was a cross-over between Buddhism and Taoism, and Chinese Ch'an Buddhism was translated into Zen in Japan.

The Confucian moral imperative promulgated the atypical Chinese respect for family and ancestors, whilst religiosity was integrated into family life and not a once-a-week observance. Some religious ceremonies, such as requiems, could be performed by Taoist, Buddhist and Muslim priests simultaneously.

We don't know much about life in the Taoist monasteries. Western encroachment upon Chinese culture resulted in the gradual downfall of religious Taoism and its temples, and the Cultural Revolution aided this in its aim of wiping out superstition, although how superstition was interpreted is a questionable matter.

Women in Taoist circles were accorded equality with men, and initiated equally in the Tao, which was not the experience in everyday society, where education for women was practically unknown. Because the female body is much more attuned to natural rhythms than the male was one reason women were venerated as being 'the body of the Tao', and Taoist masters sought to nurture the 'Inner Feminine', or Anima to use the modern equivalent. One aspect of Qi Gong is attuning the body to external temporal rhythms, as such, each of the 12 main meridians is accorded an 'energy peak' of 2 hours during the day. Other correlations of internal cycles with the days of the year and the seasons indicates how awareness of being in concert with these would lead to unity with the Tao.

The concept of harmony between opposites was figured by the Taiji or Yin/Yang symbol, understood not as static states of male/female, dark/light, night/day and so forth, but as a flow, a changing dynamic interaction of continuous movement, which is why each half of the symbol has a dot of the opposite colour in it. There is no sharp delineation between night and day; one fades gradually into the other. Like the tide washing in and out on the shore there is an alternation, or waxing and waning in events, the gravitational pull of Ch'ien and K'un, Heaven and Earth. This is covertly implied as a belief in the continuity of life, when Lao Tzu says 'The gate of heaven opens and closes'.

Yin and Yang emerged from Wu Chi, the void which prefigures existence, what in the Qabalah is represented as Ain Soph Aur or eternal limitlessness. In the Tai Chi form, when practised as a meditative reflection of the Tao, the initial state of motionless preparation is the Wu Chi stance, from which the movement commences.

The Shang Qing or Highest Purity sect practiced the process of 'Keeping the One' or 'Embracing the One', whereby union with this underlying reality would be sought by meditation and ritual or patterned behaviour, synchronising mind, breath and body. The stage known as The Return would be a state of undifferentiation between the individual and the world. 'Focus on the Centre' was another term for withdrawal. To get to this point one would pass through a period of internal observation, being aware of thoughts and feelings as they arose. This kind of insight meditation is similar to the Buddhist form, Vipassana.

The basic duality of existence is also expressed in the two strands of Taoist thought relating to the means of self-realization; the intuitive path of Wen-ta question and answer sessions offering immediate insight or 'instant enlightenment', or the way of Ts'o-ch'an or mind control, requiring the discipline of meditation. Lao Tzu and Confucius are often taken as examples of the contrary view points regarding the way to understanding. Whilst Lao Tzu's path is one of reductiveness, echoed by Agrippa as the sum of learning being vanity, the Confucian ideal is the scholar, devoted to books. Each has its own value, and each its pitfalls. The Western equivalent is the contrast between the Apollonian and Dionysian, a retreat from the world into detached contemplation, or plunging headlong into experience. Hermann Hesse's great novels 'Narziss and Goldmund' and 'The Glass Bead Game' eloquently deal with this issue. The mythical figure P'eng-tzu considered withdrawal from the world as wrong, claiming it does not impede progress to enjoy all that the world has to offer.

In actual effect the 'True Human' tends to steer a course between the two extremes of Doing and Being, recognizing the usefulness of exercise and meditation as means to an end, but not taking it too seriously. For example, a Taoist practitioner might fully engage with a session of seated meditation, but wouldn't feel duty-bound to 'endure' it and could freely walk away when bored with it without a sense of guilt.

Wu Wei is usually interpreted as 'Through doing nothing everything gets done', but it is more about not going against the natural flow of things, not trying too hard or forcing things to happen. The effortless action of the expert, bearing in mind the years of effort that can lie behind expertise in any field.

Anything that exemplifies change holds a kernel of higher truth, as nature is change. Rigid structure is unnatural. The ancient Taoists were fine observers of nature, although a Western style scientific method did not develop, because they were more concerned with insight and intuition. As it was, they arrived at the same conclusions about the world which are only now being arrived at by quantum physicists. They just didn't phrase their conclusions in formulae.

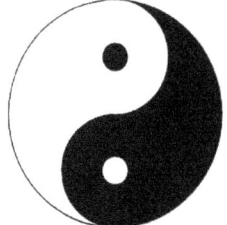
Taijitu, the well known yin/yang symbol

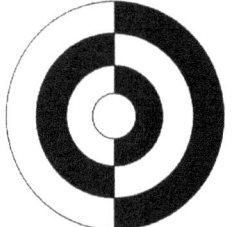
An early version

Chuang Tzu said, 'This is the principle of the supreme Tao; Chaotic!' If we take a look at Chaos Theory we find that patterns of meaning connect random phenomena. In order to show the correlation of Tao and Chaos, we'll take a brief sojourn into what is one of the most important scientific paradigms of the present.

Chaos refers both to this scientific sense of the word and to the sense of disorder that is an outcome of the Information Age we are experiencing. The speed of change, pace of life, the stresses from the wave of information we are either riding or being pulled under by, and environmental disasters, contribute to 'interesting' times, the dominion of which could be accorded to Choronzon, the demon of Dispersion, just as Chaos to the Chinese was personified by the deity Hun-tun.

Chaos Theory originated in weather prediction, and the computer modeling to that end by meteorologist Edward Lorenz in 1960. His research into apparently disordered data yielded a hidden pattern of order. The term 'The Butterfly Effect' (the idea that the flapping of a butterfly's wings could initiate atmospheric conditions that would grow exponentially, for example into a hurricane) was coined by Lorenz's discovery that a small change in an initial condition can have a drastic effect on the future result.

When Lorenz graphed his equations he got a double spiral, the Lorenz attractor. Graphs of chaotic system equations have bifurcated lines indicating order within chaos, an important characteristic that was named self-similarity. The word fractal, from fractional, is used for images conveying self-similarity. Fractal structures include blood vessels, tree branches, the lungs' internal structure and even the pattern of the heartbeat. In 'Chaos Theory and the Evolution of Consciousness and Mind: A Thermodynamic Holographic Resolution to the Mind-body Problem' by Larry R.Vandervoort, the principle of self-similarity as regarding brain-mind interrelationship is further considered in terms of consciousness evolving in a chaotic-holographic environment of algorithms or energy patterns.

A complementary principle is the holographic theory developed by the quantum physicist David Bohm and the neurophysiologist Karl Pribram. It provides an explanation for psychic phenomena and mystical experiences, as well as accounting for the idea of synchronicity and the collective unconscious. Basically the concept is that our perceived world is more or less a projection, like a hologram. Bohm theorized an implicate reality, beyond the explicate level that we are aware of. We convert the implicate frequencies by mathematical constructs, though not consciously. (I will examine this idea further in the next part of this chapter). Whereas ultimately everything is part of a whole, our observed world appears fragmented. At our local point of view we have physical bodies, but at another level, we are patterns implicated in an energy field, Bohm's quantum potential, a fundamental field pervading space and of equal potency everywhere.

It's not that the world around us is unreal; it has one reality, but there is another beyond our sensory experience. A world of frequencies and wave forms, of pure mathematics. Now by implication the recognition of synchronicities can key us into a connectivity between mind and the physical world. The involvement of consciousness in creating our reality is seriously considered by some scientists. For example, experiments by Robert G. Jahn and Brenda J. Dunne at Princeton University in 1987 provided evidence that the mind can interact psychically with the physical world.

Gardiner, Overall and Marc in the paper 'The Fractal Nature of the Brain' (NeuroQuantology, Vol.8, No.2, 2010) have written that the latest research suggests the brain's structure may be fractal. EEG data indicates a fractal dimension for the brain of between 5 and 8, which remarkably infers that it operates outside four-dimensional space-time, or in other words, in the paradigm of chaos.

This leads us to an individualistic strain of 'chaotic' research, Chaos Magic, a modern occult system created around 1976 by Peter J. Carroll and Ray Sherwin, that is results oriented, pragmatically using the techniques of science, philosophy, and any religious or ceremonial tradition that the practitioner sees as fit in order to alter one's own reality to design.

Carroll's seminal book 'Liber Null' was first published in 1978, almost ten years before James Gleick's popular explanation of Chaos Theory, 'Chaos: The Making of a New Science', appeared. Chaos Magic uses belief fluidly, changing belief systems at will in order to achieve total freedom of consciousness. One of its aims is to access the source of magical power, which is named for convenience Chaos, or just as appropriately could be called Tao. The prime method is obtaining a trance condition by motionlessness and the negation of thought, classic techniques of Taoist active meditation. There are also other means of achieving this state of gnosis.

Changing past events is one interesting theoretical area that some Chaos magicians are involved in. Again, the latest theories in mainstream science in respect to questioning the 'arrow of time' such as retrocausality and quantum entanglement, amusingly called 'spooky action at a distance' by Einstein, are not in discord with such speculation. The symbol for the system is the eight pointed Chaosphere. Chaos magic is philosophically the same as Taoism, recognizing the interrelatedness of all things in the universe and that the ultimate source of life is unbound by human attempts at anthropomorphism. The deconstruction of belief is of course a hazardous path to follow if one does not have a well grounded foundation, intellectually and emotionally.

If you consider the words themselves it is apparent Tao and Chaos are synonymous by the AO conjunction. Alpha and Omega, the beginning and end. Just to expand on my reason for preferring the Wade-Giles spelling, Tao, it is because it bears comparison to the final letter of the Hebrew alphabet (or should that be alephbeth): Tau, which is attributed to the final Major Arcana of the Tarot, The World, or more appropriately in my opinion in the Thoth/Crowley deck, the Universe, and interpreted as Completion. Incidentally, Jana Riley has observed that there is evidence the Tarot may be associated with Taoism (and again Tao is implicit in the word Tarot). The Yin/Yang symbol is notably used in the Thoth deck illustrations, and Aleister Crowley considered Taoist Masters as the highest form of adepts, as he wrote in his novel 'Moonchild'.

II. THE NUMBER EIGHT:

A Case Study of Pattern Significance.

'Everything is in relation to everything else'. The Buddha

There is chaos, and there is a grand unifying thread through its maze; the recurring number. Number is a means of investigating and understanding everything possible to be known, to paraphrase Pico della Mirandola in his Mathematical Conclusions. Number fixes time and space through co-ordinates. Max Tegmark of MIT thinks the universe actually is maths. A mathematical structure that we are just revealing rather than a science we devise. With regard to Taoist practice the continual recurrence of the same number is due to a recognition, whether conscious or through covert perception, of a resonant harmonious pattern being established through the body.

As we connect with a sense of underlying order, synchronicities become more frequent. This is effected because the root of the matter is our immersion in a grand code, the binary expression that underlies creation. As the basis of reality is numerical pattern it is interesting to find that certain numbers have been accorded significance by a variety of cultures throughout time. One very striking example is the number 8.

A Fibonacci number and the symbol of infinity when placed on its side, the 'lemniscate of infinitude' (lovely term), to the Chinese it expresses the totality of the universe. The word in the Chinese language for 8 is 'ba', which sounds similar to the word for wealth or prosper. Therefore 888 is considered particularly lucky. The opening ceremony of the Summer Olympics in Beijing was at eight minutes and eight seconds past eight p.m. local time on 8/8/08. Many of the exercises of Qi Gong are arranged in groups of eight; the eight Yuan Qi exercises, the 'Eight Pieces of Brocade', and so on. There are eight trigrams, which are related through Confucian idealism to the family unit; Father, Mother, three sons and three daughters. Taoist deities include the eight Immortals, the Ba Hsien. Eight is classed as a Yin number (odd numbers are Yang, even Yin).

Since eight is the first cubic number (there are eight vertices in a cube), it can represent the earth. There are eight directions to the compass. As a representation of the totality of the space/time continuum, the 4 dimensions are added to the 2 solstices and 2 equinoxes. The pagan eight-fold wheel of the year celebrates 8 festivals.

In Babylon, Egypt and Arabia it was a number with a sun association. The solar disk was decorated with eight rays. To the Egyptians, it represented balance and cosmic harmony. The god Thoth had eight disciples. For the ancient Greeks, the number was dedicated to Dionysus, born on the eighth month of the year. As a symbol of 'the Cosmic Christ' it expresses new life and resurrection, matter and incarnation, and according to Clement of Alexandria, Christ places under the sign of eight the one he made to be born again.

Through the Qabalistic formulation of Gematria, converting letters into a numerical value, the word Qeshet, Rainbow (the sign of the covenant given to Noah after the Flood) = 800, which is also the value of the Greek words Lord and Faith. And incidentally the value of the final letter of the Greek alphabet, Omega. Connecting Hebrew and Greek is a central doctrine of the Church. Thus, Jesus in Greek (Iesous) and The Salvation of our God in Hebrew (Yeshoth Elohenu) = 800, the number of transcendence. Qeshet guph, incidentally, is the 'rainbow body', the ascension form (reference this to the spectrum of colours of the Chakras).

To the Cabalists the Temple of Jerusalem had eight gates; the eighth would only open for the Messiah. Circumcision as a sign of the Covenant was to be performed on the eighth day. Hanukah lasts eight days and eight nights.

One of the first times I noticed an eight-pointed star in a specifically Christian religious setting was on the floor of the Mary chapel in Wells Cathedral. The Christian view of it is as a symbol of regeneration and baptism, so baptismal fonts usually have an octagonal base. There were eight people on the Ark who emerged from the Flood waters, a fundamental baptismal moment. The eight -point star, known as the Star of Redemption, is connected to other 'Queens of Heaven' apart from Mary, such as the Sumerian goddess Inanna and the Babylonian Ishtar, or Astarte, and is an emblem of the Ogdoadic Tradition derived from the mystery religions of the Mediterranean and the Hermetic and Neoplatonic Schools. On Mesopotamian cuneiform tablets the eight pointed star was a determinative sign indicating 'deity' (see Jaynes, 'The Origin of Consciousness in the Breakdown of the Bicameral Mind', p.185).

In Buddhism, there are eight Paths to Perfection, eight symbols of long life, and eight degrees of monk. The lotus is symbolised with eight petals. The Noble Eightfold Path is represented by the Dharmachakra, or Wheel of Law, taken as a general symbol for Buddhism. In Hinduism, there are eight forms of Shiva, illustrated by eight lingams laid out around a central one, and the yogi Patanjali devised eight 'limbs' or sutras.

Although the usual number of major Chakras or energy centres of esoteric anatomy is 7, some sources locate an eighth, the Chakra of the Soul or Star Chakra, above the Crown. You may find eight-pointed stars in Moroccan textile patterns and in architectural detail, also in Islam where it represents the Seal of the Prophets. Islamic salat practice has eight postures. The number eight is similarly of importance in Sufism.

Pythagoras suggested a Law of Octaves, and Nikolai Tesla also believed in a Law of Eight. The chemical elements in the Periodic Table fall into eight families.

As Pluto was disqualified as a planet in 2006 by the International Astronomical Union's redefinition (it's now designated by a number, 134340), we are defined cosmologically by being positioned in a planetary octave, from Mercury to Uranus (Ouranos being a particularly potent focus for some forms of magical work).

The multiple 8X8 has also many resonances. There are 64 days between the Hebrew festivals of Purim and Lag B'Omer, 64 petals on the lotus that represents the Ajna Chakra or Third Eye point, 64 squares on a chess board, 64 codons in the DNA structure and 64 hexagrams in the I Ching.

The last two correspondences have been the subject of a remarkable study by Katya

The Gate of Gifts: Aspects of Esotericism

Walter, 'Tao of Chaos'. The genetic code's 64 codons are composed of four different molecules, base nucleotides, that are arranged in a combination of triplets. Walter demonstrates that the DNA code and the I Ching have a fascinating correlation - the bonding of gene base pairs and the equivalent bonding of lines in the hexagrams. She presents an extensive thesis on this coding correspondence including a comparative cross-referencing of hexagram meanings and amino acid properties, and further analysis right down to atomic level.

Her research offers a theoretical explanation for such phenomena as synchronicity and the origin of divinatory systems that have a basis in the number eight, including the I Ching, the Runes and the Tarot, which some researchers consider to have a core of eight Major Arcana cards, the remainder of the pack being elaborations of these (the Fool, Magician, High Priestess, Emperor, Empress, Heirophant, Hermit and Star). Divinatory systems momentarily occupy or distract the rational critical mind, allowing access to deep levels of consciousness. Within some of the major methods, namely those mentioned above, there are several points of commonality, as on reflection could be expected.

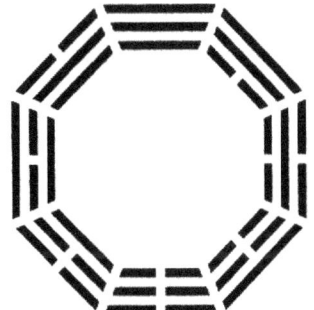
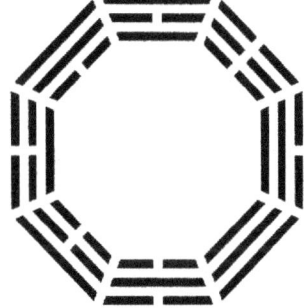

Fu Hsi early heaven arrangement   *The King Wen Later heaven arrangement*

Fu Hsi, one of the mythical Five Emperors of China, is credited with the discovery of the I Ching. There are two diagrams portraying the arrangement of the trigrams - the Fu Hsi or H'sien Tien (Early or Pre-Heaven) arrangement, and the King Wen or Hou Tien (Late or Post-Heaven). The symbols were, as legend has it, seen upon the backs of a turtle and then a dragon horse. The latter is an intriguing conflation of a creature, probably representative of Yin/Yang duality.

The first arrangement denotes polar opposites and the Void, the second depicts development in time and space. From the eight trigrams, by combining pairs of them there evolved the hexagrams, and from this came the eight multiplied by eight pattern of the I Ching. This seems to represent the ground pattern of the universe in a very primal manner; as has been observed there are 64 squares on the board of that archetypal 'Battleground of Life' game, chess.

The famous Sinologist Joseph Needham believed that chess, or the early Indian version of Chaturanga, evolved from a Chinese divinatory technique for determining Yin/Yang balance in relation to military strategy (there is a view that all board games are derived from divination methods). The chessboard squares as coloured black and white similarly represent Yin and Yang polarity. As for the 16 pieces on each side, Jung's original model of eight personality types has been doubled by the Myers Briggs Type Indicator to 16, and the 16 Court cards of the Tarot are taken to represent the personality. There are also 16 'Golden' hexagrams forming the core of the I Ching.

It can be noted that the standard model of elementary particles, representing the 'building blocks' of the universe, is composed of 6 quarks, 6 leptons and 4 force-carrying particles; 16. The physiological integrity of the number eight is observed in such conditions as there being an octave mapping of neurons in the auditory thalamus of the brain. Perhaps this is the reason we have an octave scale in music.

So my point in following through this thread of numerical connectivity is to establish that it's reasonable to infer an embodiment of pure number at an intense level creating resonances in the external world, what we may call Pattern Significance. Of course this is open to the accusation of delusions of reference or apophenia, seeing meaningful patterns in meaningless data, and that you might take any number and find significance in it; I'm particularly drawn to the number eight as my family configuration happens to conform to the Confucian ideal associated with the Ba Gua Trigram arrangement; Parents, 3 sons, 3 daughters. And although I'm not a follower of Astrology, I was born under the eighth house, Scorpio ('oh, you must have a sting in your tail'. If I've heard that once…).

Beyond the pink glow of solipsism I feel there is an inherent truth, a case to be made for number as the relational nexus between the abstract and concrete worlds. The Tables of Correspondences, the Doctrine of Signatures that was created in the Middle Ages as a map for Sympathetic Magic, these attempts at drawing diverse elements together do not appear so incongruous in light of Chaos Theory's proposition that all things are interconnected.

It can be fairly observed that our Information Age is founded upon number, the binary units 0 and 1, which if considered purely as symbols are naturally very relevant, the circle and the straight line. It's said there are two Ways to enlightenment, the upright and the averse; 'Be as a flame or a still pool of water'. An interesting recent development is the Quantum computer, that can integrate the binary units. Ordinary computers compute with 1 and 0, but the quantum computer bit can be 1 and 0 at the same time. That is perhaps an apposite signification for our current collective condition.

III. THE WESTERN ESOTERIC TRADITION

'The Framing of this circle on the ground
Brings whirlwinds, tempests, thunder and lightning'. Dr. Faustus, Marlowe.

There is a kind of contemporary assault on secrecy, where all secrets are regarded as being inherently bad. An outcome of the present predilection for a lack of boundaries. But people who can't separate themselves from the cacophony of the times are subject to automatism, becoming shadows of their true selves. We need some separation and containment in order to establish our own unique identity and commune with it; this is portrayed as the setting up of an Inner Temple. Seclusion is important but becoming ever harder to find both externally and internally in the 'open' society. When things become commonplace they are apt to lose their power, so it is not always elitism in keeping some secrets. This is a matter of spiritual security.

To give a very basic overview of the West's 'History of Secrets':

The word Esoteric comes from the Greek esoterikos, meaning 'belonging to an inner circle', and originally applied to Pythagorean doctrines. Plato and Aristotle first used the terms esoteric and exoteric in reference to knowledge. The Academy they taught in was to begin with a grove or circle of olive trees, hence the inference of an 'inner circle' receiving higher education.

The term coined by one of the founders of the Golden Dawn magical order, Samuel Liddel Macgregor Mathers, at the end of the 19th century to describe Western as opposed to Eastern occult teachings, was 'The Western Mystery Tradition'. This covers a wide range of knowledge, both magical and religious, proceeding from the ancient world and the systems of Egyptian and Hellenic religion, including the Greek Eleusinian and Orphic Schools, taking in Middle Eastern Zoroastrianism, Gnosticism and the teachings of the Essenes and the Jewish mystics. Within the study itself there is an exoteric aspect, the historical record of which has been traced by scholars such as Frances Yates, and the esoteric practices themselves.

Oddly enough the Western esoteric tradition's studies actually flourished inside the monastic orders, particularly the Benedictine. Such adepts of alchemy as the German Abbot Trithemius and Basilius Valentinus were Benedictines. Edward Kelly, accomplice of Dr. Dee, was alleged to have obtained an alchemical substance from the Benedictine Abbey of Glastonbury. As a parallel, Chinese spiritual practices also largely derive from a monastic background.

In the Middle Ages Spain hosted the Catholic, Islamic and Jewish faiths with relative equanimity. The Sephardic Jews developed the Qabalah mystical system, which became integrated with Neoplatonism and was Christianized during the Renaissance by Pico della Mirandola and Johannes Reuchlin. The angelic conjurations of Agrippa and Dee were products of Christian Qabalism, and alchemy was a supplement to these endeavours.

Rosicrucianism might also be seen as an offshoot of this 'alternative' religious movement, and during the Enlightenment there arose the Freemasonic and Rosicrucian Brotherhoods, precursors of the Illuminati conspiracy theory elite.

In the 19th century Madame Helena Blavatsky caused a schism through incorporating Eastern methods such as Yoga into her Theosophy, whilst one of the most important magical societies of all time, the Hermetic Order of the Golden Dawn, developed its own rituals and system of initiation that would prove to be extremely influential.

As mentioned, the term 'The Western Mystery Tradition' being formulated as such at this time, it was seen to a degree as a localized expression of 'The Matter of Britain', therefore focusing on Celtic mythology, the Grail Quest, the conjectural elevation of the Druids. Other terms include 'The Perennial Philosophy', 'The Inner Way' and the 'Esoteric Tradition'.

Out of these disparate subjects there are clear comparisons to Taoist inner work in the major areas of: Magical Ritual with its associated patterns of symbolic movement and gesture; the dual traditions of alchemy; complementary numerical and divinatory systems; and magical/philosophical conceptions of the universe. It does not require a leap of imagination to find an affinity within these main methods of the spiritual quest. Obviously, as such terms as Esotericism and Mystery Tradition have Greek and Latin roots, there is not a literal equivalent in Chinese terms; also there is a difference in the historical and societal climates affecting the dissemination of such knowledge. The studies in themselves though certainly yield points of equivalence.

The precepts of magic for example are close to Tao. As I noted in the foreword, magical practice is a relevant and contemporary part of Taoism, with three major sects, the Mao-shan, Celestial Teachers and Kun-Lun involved in magical rituals. The comparatively neglected, very influential writer W.G. Gray was instrumental in making inferred analogies between Taoist ideas and Western magical technique, as in expressing the importance of the experience of Nothingness (as it's said 'Let nothing be before God', Gray proposed 'Let us therefore worship Nothing', and condensed this radical thought with his Omnil formulation).

The magical effecting of willed change is commonly associated with ritual correspondence. Through appropriate robes, incense and ritual gesture within a circumscribed space, the magic circle, the magician seeks unification with archetypal energies by utilising a sympathetic resonance to impress the subconscious and separate the mind from the mundane level. This is the same rationale behind higher aspects of the Taoist energetic syllabus. It could be likened to psychodrama, the method in humanistic psychology for 'acting out' processes. Or indeed, simply drama, a performance on a stage that bears meaning to those involved. Martial arts forms or katas and Qi Gong sets are in effect magic rituals, because they 'effect willed change', and as such have a property of facilitating connection to higher aspects of consciousness. Taoists often create their own rituals without the use of a priest as an intermediary.

Essentially, TAO is the symbolic basis for the Western Magical Ritual Tradition, if you think of the T as the Cross, A as an incipient pentagram and O the magic circle. When, as the Taoists tend to, you recognize the sacred in the mundane, then it is unnecessary to separate magic from our everyday experience of the world. As a character in the TV show 'True Blood' put it: 'Magic is intention and energy'.

It remains to be seen if there is any longer a value in the attribution 'East/West', in the sense that it has long been used to define philosophical outlooks or spiritual practices. The perception of a global divide has been likened to the right and left hemispheres of the brain, whereby it is usually posited that the East has operated from a position of holism akin to right brain functioning and the West is predominantly left-brain biased (overtly rational, valuing logic over intuition, and so forth). This segregation, it may be construed, has been decidedly breached by the Information Revolution with synthesis the corollary of our smaller world. Coincidentally we are reaching a point where the magnetic poles are due to flip as occurs every few thousand years. Our coordinates are literally shifting.

The psyche, as Jung pointed out, has a common level for all of us, whatever our ethnic background or upbringing. The symbols and motifs of the collective unconscious are accessible by anyone, which provides a key to realising the particular utility of the Taoist path both as a discipline unto itself and as a way that meets common ground with others.

That is not to devalue the origins of traditions. It is essential to maintain an understanding of inherited wisdom, the lineage of real knowledge. The quality of such teaching lies in the parameters it provides, its clear lines of guidance. Without a direct, verifiable line of genealogy, words can obfuscate and become mere dogma, or else meld into a weak confusion if not bolstered by a foundation. The occultist Dion Fortune, writing in the 1930s, was concerned that people did not lose track of the native esoteric traditions into which they were born. In fact she advised against the adoption of foreign practices. Her concerns were understandable, but 80 years on the world has integrated cultures and blended beliefs, if only to a certain extent. There is still separation and differentiation, even though it leads at times to outright prejudice and narrow minds. Traditional methods and paths best serve us when we can tap into their collective energy, impelling us forward as a motivational force rather than stultifying or imprisoning in artificial constraint.

We should bear in mind that we interpret teachings from other cultures through the medium of our own experience. I was told of an English Tai Chi teacher who was so desperate to inhabit the identity of the Chinese that he learnt the language fluently, began to eat only Chinese food and dressed in Chinese clothes constantly. There is such a thing as going too far. My first Wing Chun teacher was a chain-smoker who even had a cigarette in his mouth as he taught (avoiding being branded by it was a lesson in itself). I may have wished to emulate his martial ability but that didn't mean smoking 60 cigarettes a day.

With the dissemination of a broader outlook in magical culture, the Golden Dawn/Crowleyan/Qabalah-influenced paradigm is just one path amongst many; a whole world of various traditions yields undoubtedly a mine of comparable practices. As always, finding the middle path, 'the crossing place where we meet' to quote the greatly missed Robert Holdstock, is an essential goal for our bemused times.

IV. COMPARATIVE ALCHEMY

The Schools of Wai Dan and Nei Dan, External and Internal alchemy, arose during the 3rd century AD, roughly the same time as the emergence of the art in Alexandria, where it was associated with Hermes-Thoth, or Thrice Greatest Hermes, Hermes Trismegistus (from whom also we obtain Hermeticism). Joseph Needham has noted that originally the word Alchemy was of Taoist origin, predating the Arabic interpretation.

It was perhaps more biased toward metallurgy in the West and pursuing the means of effecting the transmutation of base materials into gold, although Roger Bacon in the 13th century was involved in both this aspect and the acquisition of long life, and Paracelsus used the study medically.

In China the early alchemists combined experimenting with compounds and elixirs with meditation and exercise techniques. One of the most important texts of Taoist alchemy was the Tsan-tung-chi or Union of the Triplex Equation, by Wei Po-yang. The Internal School was responsible for the idea of inner cultivation and the development of Qi. By about the 11th century, however, the practices had become debased and stagnated. A new philosophical synthesis of mind and body grew around the same time as the three major systems of Taoism, Buddhism and Confucianism merged.

Laboratory-based alchemy tangentially produced such discoveries as gunpowder, medicines and techniques of smelting metals, thereby developing in one direction into chemistry. There was also a metaphorical aspect as commented upon by Jung. What then was phrased as transformation of gross matter (lead) into gold was a symbol for the refining of one's raw nature and the attainment of immortality. Many Taoist alchemists, including Ko Hung (284-364 AD) compiled teachings on immortality and its achievement. Another famous writer of texts on internal alchemy was Chang Po-tuan, a major lineage holder of the Complete Reality School. The actual ingestion of substances in pursuit of this aim, such as mercury and arsenic, often led to the realization of spiritual liberation sooner than expected, although there is a debate about whether the experimenters were in fact aware of the poisonous nature of what they were dealing with and were trying to administer beneficial amounts without overdosing. Therefore the deaths would still have been accidental but not entirely through ignorance. After centuries of failure in achieving physical immortality the meaning of the term began to be redefined, and during the Sung dynasty such components as furnace, cauldron, fire and water were used as metaphors for internal processes. The consumption of symbolic substances to achieve transmutation is dramatized in the Catholic Mass where the congregation is invited to partake of the Sacrament, the Body of Christ (a Solar deity, the Sacrificed God). Magical ritual is a living component of the Church.

One example of the blending of physical alchemical research with a more conceptual approach is the naming of the Dan Tien, which translates as Elixir Field, or Field of Cinnabar, cinnabar being an important alchemical substance. The Three Elixir Fields, psycho-spiritual energy centres in the body, were first conceived in the Huangting Jing, the Yellow Court Classic, a product of the Shangqing (Supreme Purity) Taoist tradition of the Tang period.

To the Taoists, the world is quintessentially real, an extension of Tao, and by following the principle of balance one could prolong life. The body was not something to be denied, but a vehicle for expression.

'Journey to the West', the fable about the Monkey King, ruler of a nation but not of himself, has an alchemical theme. After becoming involved in causing all manner of trouble, Taoist immortals attempt to put him through an alchemical spiritual training by placing him in a cauldron of eight trigrams, but he escapes, only to be imprisoned in the material world. He is eventually freed by the goddess of compassion, Kuan Yin, the Queen of Heaven who was originally a male deity, Avalokitesvara. Tracing the etymology of the Sanskrit root of this name is an interesting exercise as we find Avallach/Avalon and associations with apples which is unfortunately outside the scope of this study, except to mention the apple as an obvious symbol with multiple layers of meaning, including the attainment of immortality. I will make further reference to the intriguing transformation of Kuan Yin in the chapter on the Te.

The cauldron reference is also notable as analogous to the cauldrons in Celtic myth that have their own transformative roles to play. The Dan Tien are figuratively known as cauldrons, the general symbolism being the interplay of fire and water to produce some other material or state. Li and Kan, Fire and Water, are represented as the Middle and Lower Dan Tien which are activated to produce, in essence, the Philosopher's

Stone, a mysterious object or material which acted as a catalyst for transformation. The ancient formula, Dissolve and Solidify, Solve et Coagula, was a principle also embraced by the Yin/Yang duality where Yang is the Dissolving aspect and Yin the Solidifying. The formula is also expressed in a colourful way by the famous dictum: 'Visit the Interior parts of the Earth; By Rectification shall you find the Hidden Stone'. Visita Interiora Terrae Rectificando Invenies Occultum Lapidem, or Vitriol, the alchemical universal solvent.

There are ten alchemical stages of the 'Chemical Marriage' enumerated in the 17th century text the Rosarium Philosophorum, the Philosopher's Rose Garden, which could be taken to complement the ten sephiroth of the Tree of Life. A body of knowledge sometimes being referred to as a garden, the Qabalah is known as a 'Garden of Pomegranates', another fruit associated with immortality (as well as the myth of Persephone and as a representation of fecundity). The stages are:

1. The Mercurial Fountain. This is the disintegrated state. Mercury or Mercurius is the medium that integrates opposites.

2. The King and Queen. The union of one's being , the bringing together of anima and animus.

3. Assimilating the Shadow.

4. Descent into Water. The Nekyia or night-sea journey.

5. The Coniunctio. The conjunction that conceives the lapis or philosopher's stone.

6. The Nigredo, the Dark Night of the Soul.

7. The Ascent of the Soul.

8. Purification.

9. The Return of the Soul.

10. Rebirth into the Unus Mundus, the One World.

These stages are collectively analogous to the Taoist alchemical progression of dissolution, union, ascent and return. Ritual initiations held by groups working with the model of the Qabalistic Tree are similarly designed on a basis of climbing extra-sensory levels and returning to the mundane, bringing the newly acquired consciousness-shift with you.

The three vital alchemical substances, a principle formulated by Paracelsus in the

West, are Sulphur, Salt and Mercury which are equivalent in Hindu thought to the three Gunas, the forces within prakriti or existence; Rajas (active force), Tamas (passive) and Sattvas (the balancing energy).

The process of Separation, Purification and Recombination is symbolised by the three elements of Fire (=Sulphur), Air (=Mercury) and Water (=Salt). These combine to form Earth (just to clarify, this is entirely metaphorical and not related to actual manifest elements). Sulphur is Yang, Mercury Yin, and Salt the Union. Prenatal energy is the energy of Water, Postnatal energy is Fire energy.

The three key elements are also incidentally associated (by the curious attribution of meaning to each letter of the Hebrew alphabet) with the three 'Mother' Letters of Aleph, Mem and Shin, standing consecutively for Air, Water and Fire. There is a complementary formula of the letters Cheth, Resh and Mem but I refer the reader to Hall's 'The Secret Teachings of All Ages' for further elucidation on this point, only to mention here that Cheth, the 8th letter in the Hebrew alphabet, is attributed to The Chariot in the Tarot, and that the Qabalah was derived from the Maaseh Merkabah, the Workings of the Chariot, which in turn refers to Ezekiel's Vision. Cheth means Fence, implying enclosure, containment; the Temenos or sacred precinct.

Aleph or Air is a balancing medium between the active and passive principles of Fire and Water. In the Five Element system it can be represented by both Wood (=Spirit) and Metal. Trees actually grow more from the influence of air than of earth, and the metal sword is a symbol of air/intellect in the way of discernment, the mind being used to cut away illusions.

So, as I've shown, the formula of Internal Taoist alchemy that makes use of the elements by techniques of Nei Gong are similarly a method of Qabalistic alchemy. How did such dissimilar cultures arrive at the same formulation of using element symbols to signify inner processes? Synchronous deep introspection and a correspondent realization of an ultimate truth is probably the only conclusion to be drawn, failing any evidence of cultural transaction.

The pursuit of physical immortality is by any standard a questionable activity, because considering its actual attainment the state would entail intense isolation; loss of family and friends and a complete separation from the mass of humanity. Psychologically it could be mooted as just a basic fear of death, a fear that this world is all there is. Or a rebellion against nature, as contrary to the obvious fact that life is in a continual flux of change, it advocates a condition of changelessness. It would in fact be necessary to become other than human hearted, which as we previously have noted is a quality of the Tao. Yet there is still a contemporary pursuit of the same goal, as in Rebirthing (see 'Physical Immortality' by Leonard Orr and Sondra Ray), the work of Robert Coon, as a theme in science fiction and fantasy writing (Robert Silverberg's entertaining 'The

Book of Skulls') and the continuing glamour of vampires. A strange book called 'Bible of the Undead' presents a method for attaining physical immortality (allegedly), but I would say the participant would need to be a very balanced, self-aware person to follow what is proposed. Another engrossing study is 'The Book of Gnostic Revelation'.

There is a technical difference between immortality and extending the lifespan; immortal life suggests being capable of avoiding the 'thousand natural shocks that flesh is heir to', such as the inevitable higher incidence of accidents occurring, even if the body did not age. However, an extended or indefinite lifespan is seriously considered a viable achievement of future medical advances in such areas as genetic engineering and molecular nanotechnology, with its development of cellular repair machines.

While the emphasis is now on a symbolic, psychological interpretation, there are a few modern alchemists working with their own laboratories. In the broader context of making change, any transformation of a base condition into a more idealised one can be considered an alchemical action.

Alchemy lives and breathes.

3. QI GONG

DEFINING QI

Qi Gong (pronounced Chee Gung) translates as Energy Work. It is differentiated from Nei Gong or Inner Work usually by the linking of conscious breathing with physical movements, breath becoming a medium for the realisation of Qi, whereas Nei Gong practices are more a case of working from the inside out as it were, often entailing still postures and meditation, the direct experience of life energy without necessarily a concentration on the breath.

A dictionary definition of energy, the one that science likes to adhere to, is simply 'the capacity to do work'. It is understandable that the scientists in our culture are derisive of any interpretation of energy that deviates from their own. Precision in terms is essential, and the general decline in standards of literacy in favour of 'freedom of expression' leads to unclear thinking. We can't, after all, express ourselves and manifest our aims without the underlying structure of a functional grammar.

With the gradual progression of new techniques in the chemical analysis of biological material, the need for a vital force to explain life was made apparently insupportable. But as Ernst Mayr, the evolutionary biologist, has pointed out, though the interaction of components in a holistic pattern must be understood by analysis, that does not mean the mechanistic model of the human organism is validated.

On the contrary, the Western scientific community can no longer substantiate an argument against the holistic view of energy even though the scientific method is not amenable to theories of bio-energy. We are all fundamentally, and at the core particle/wave function level, composed energetically, as is everything around us. So the employment of the word may jar to the Victorian analytical viewpoint, but I have to subscribe to its use in describing what are after all abstract states. An alternative term would only similarly be subject to criticism.

Of course the whole arena of complementary therapy and psycho-spiritual exercise is open to accusations of pseudoscience and magical thinking (as it is unfortunately applied in its derogatory sense). The essential question, though, should be whether a practice contributes to overall wellbeing. There have been attempts to place the concept of Qi on an 'acceptable' basis. In the 1980s the Chinese government were keen to promote their heritage, and twenty years earlier, responding to a World Health Organization directive, had created TCM, Traditional Chinese Medicine. Perhaps a better translation would be Traditional Communist Medicine, as the components were arbitrarily selected by a group of committee physicians. TCM is not the totality it appears to be, but a fragment. Consider the size of the country. Different forms of medicine evolved over the centuries in each village and province. So as Qi Gong was promoted, some Chinese scientists tried to placate Western analysts by suggesting Qi was a metaphor. Naturally, actual physical structures cannot be found that correlate to such models as the Qi Meridians, although there has been a great deal of research into measuring energy fields in and around the human body, such as the images of an aura captured by the Russian scientist Semyon Davidich Kirlian in the 1920s, a method subsequently named Kirlian photography. Another example is the documentation of energy points made in the 1990s that related to the acupuncture points, using a device known as the SQUID (superconducting quantum interference device), an extremely sensitive magnetometer used to measure weak magnetic fields. This has led some researchers to equate Qi with the idea of a quantum field effect.

The paper published in the Winter 2001 edition of the American Journal of Chinese Medicine, 'Evidence of Qi Gong Energy and its Biological Effect on the Enhancement of the Phagocytic Activity of Human Polymorphonuclear Leukocytes' by Fukushima, Kataoka, Hamada and Matsumoto, presented evidence that in a controlled, independently monitored experiment, a phosphate buffered saline solution was treated by a Qi Gong master and found to influence cellular activity. As similar effects were produced by microwave irradiation and infrared laser pulse treatment, Qi might be compared to these levels of energy.

Results can be erratic in cold-testing conditions; research into the efficacy of acupuncture does not always take into account the capability of the practitioner. Traditionally acupuncturists spent years training in Qi Gong before they even began using the needles. In contrast to this, the Medical Acupuncture Society was founded by Felix Mann, who didn't believe in the idea of meridians or even the traditional acupuncture points, and yet has still created a fully functional curative methodology.

This leads one to consider the view of the respected martial artist Tim Cartmell, who thinks Intention, or 'Yi', is more essential, and that it is really not that important whether Qi exists or not. 'Where the mind goes, Qi flows' is another of those ubiquitous Chinese sayings. So although Qi is most popularly related to the breath it can be interpreted as life force, mental focus or in terms of an electrochemical effect. I tend toward an explanation in terms of vitality, which is something most people can relate to.

HISTORY, STYLES AND EFFECTS.

The origins of Qi Gong may extend as far back as around 2700 BC and Huang Ti, the legendary Yellow Emperor. He was said to have practiced Dao Yin, a form of exercise which translates as 'guiding (or leading) energy'. The exercises could have come from ancient shamanic rites and magical dance patterns. In the 2nd century AD Hua Tuo produced the 'Movement of the Five Animals Set', or 'Five Animal Frolics'. Ko Hung the alchemist had an 18 movement form, and Da Mo or Bodhidharma as he was originally known before he arrived in China developed a set of exercises for the monks of the Shaolin Temple to strengthen their bodies so they could remain seated in meditation for longer periods of time. These were collected as the famous Tendon Changing and Marrow Cleansing Classics (Yi Chin Ching and Hsi Sui Ching).

During the boom in interest in Qi Gong in the 1980s, the Falun Gong movement emerged, extolling a synthesis of Buddhist and Taoist principles. The vast number of practitioners in this school (estimated at 70 million by the end of the 1990s) attracted the attention of the authorities. After peaceful protests against unfair media coverage, Falun Gong was banned by the Communist Party in 1999.

Many cultures throughout the ages have had a concept of internal energy, or life force. It's even there in our modern rendering of heroic myth, 'Star Wars'. The Japanese equivalent is Ki, and to the Hindus it's Prana, or the Serpent Power, Kundalini. The Qabalists have Chiah.

Aristotle and Hippocrates thought of pneuma, or breath, as the spirit of life. George Stahl, court physician to Frederick William 1 of Prussia, conceived of the anima as life force. Then there is Hans Driesch's Vitalist theory, the elan vital, Carl Reichenbach's idea of Odic force, Franz Anton Mesmer's 'animal magnetism', Wilhelm Reich's Orgone Energy, the ideas of Vril and the Norse Aethm, and Native American Indian and Shamanic equivalents.

There are innumerable styles and forms of Qi Gong. Some work very closely with the medical models of the meridians, yin/yang polarity and the Wu Xing or Five Element theory. Others are gentle stretching exercises that work the muscles and joints. There are exercises that can be prescribed for specific ailments, and others designed for the development of martial art ability. Then there are Buddhist and Confucian styles as well as the Taoist ones.

Where Western exercise tends to exert stress upon the muscular and circulatory/respiratory systems, such as jogging, gymnasium work-outs, sports and aerobics, Qi Gong works on a subtle and seemingly indirect way of improving physical function by such means as adjusting structural alignment and taking into account the whole pattern of individual constitution, strengths, weaknesses and tendencies. So there is a more gradual improvement in well-being, as the body adjusts itself from old habitual patterns, but there is the benefit that the exercises can be continued well into old age, unlike the more strenuous popular forms of physical activity. Instead of exerting muscular contraction the emphasis is upon muscular relaxation, and energy generation rather than energy expenditure. It might seem paradoxical but a feeling of strength is not what is aimed for in Qi exercise, rather a whole body sensation of loose effortless power, or connectedness.

The general effect of Qi Gong exercise is benefit to the cardiovascular, lymphatic and nervous systems and increased muscular and tendon strength. There is also evidence that it works at a very deep level to enhance the immune system and improve cellular and bone health improvement can be irregular instead of an even progress as blocks in internal states of energy are released. There can even be an initial worsening of some symptoms as the body adjusts itself to improved functioning. It is as if the body has its own consciousness; it can rebel unexpectedly or send messages to us, as when we eat something that isn't really good for us. When the psychosomatic condition of the habitual 'comfort zone' is altered then there will be a settling-in period, and the essential thing is to persist. The mind pervades the body, and is not merely constrained to the head. At least, that is an alternative perception, after a few centuries of Cartesian duality.

The detoxifying stage of Qi Gong may even result in emotions unexpectedly arising. In this case one should consider it as energy patterns being released in order to facilitate a more balanced internal state of health.

In fact Chinese medicine has the somewhat startling concept (to a modern Western view) that the internal organs each have their own form of consciousness (although the same idea is found in early Greek philosophy). This is rather a metaphor to create a new way of being aware of the inner aspect of health, usually neglected by a facile concentration on the outer appearance of the body. As, on awaking in the morning it is advised not to rush out of bed too soon because the heart may still be asleep. To quote Jaynes again, 'Consciousness has no location except as we imagine it has' (op. cit., p.46).

After a while the practitioner does actually become more aware of the 'feeling' of an inner homeostasis. It is obviously not a cure-all; each individual has to evaluate their own state of health or lack of it in terms of an over-all picture including life-style, diet, environment, relationships, work, and habits. The hyperbole found in some Chinese produced books on the subject may be the result of mistranslation or due to an over-zealous desire to impress. Sometimes the claims are quite entertaining and belong more to the world of Chinese theatre, such as masters emitting light from their hands; that would certainly be a useful ability for the times I've come back from the pub on a moonless night and struggled to fit the door key in the lock.

The foundation of Taoist Qi Gong is simple to summarise; it entails Sitting, Standing and Walking. Admittedly there is some elaboration upon these acts, but it could be said they relate to the three powers (san cai) of Heaven, Mankind and Earth, and the three treasures (san bao) of Essence, Spirit and Qi (there is a similar triune doctrine in the Dzogchen lineage of Buddhism; Essence, Nature and Energy). Heaven (Ch'ien) is Yang energy, Earth (K'un) is Yin (as in Mother Earth), and we are balanced in between (Jen, human). Our Jing, essence, is stored in the kidneys and relates to the pre-birth experience, the Waters of Life when we were suspended in the amniotic fluid. Qi Gong and Tai Chi are said to enhance kidney energy in particular, the kidneys being the receptacles of inherited energy. Our postnatal acquired energy, which we can build up, is Qi. Shen, our Spirit, interpenetrates the physical body; it is within us and also surrounding us like the idea of an aura.

We start from the initial point of stillness that is known as Wu Chi, or The Void, a meditative or empty state of potential from which all our actions originate. It is necessary to be empty before we can fully receive anything. An empty' mind allows us to sense energy blocks in the body, respond instinctively in the martial arts, and open a spiritual awareness. This is followed by Prenatal Energy, the spark of life, our essential inheritance. Postnatal Energy is the form of vitality that we acquire and control in our daily activity, including our connection with others and the

The only way to experience the effectiveness of Qi Gong is to do it, to balance theory with practice. Chinese students traditionally didn't question what they were taught;

they just followed instruction. Thinking too much blocks the Qi! When we become truly involved, we forget ourselves and find spontaneous action and effortless activity, Wu Wei. It's said that 'Breathing means to empty oneself and wait for Tao'.

Al-Ghazzali, the Persian philosopher of the 11th century, noted that theory is far different from practice, that a state of transport to mystical perception is incommunicable to the discursive method of science.

4. THE HEALTH CLASSIC

The Neijing, also known as the Yellow Emperor's Classic, is a remarkable Taoist text positing an integrative interpretation of health as being holistically connected with environment. What it stated some 4000 years ago is a truth that modern civilisation is belatedly realising; we are inseparable from nature. Only now that science is arriving at the same conclusion of indivisibility, as contrasting to the piecemeal fragmented view of the Aristotelian method, is the genius of these ancient masters being appreciated.

The basis of diagnosis is the Wu Xing or Five Element Theory, and the balance of Yin and Yang in accord with Western medicine's concept of Homeostasis, the maintenance and regulation of a stable internal state. The various biological components involved in this dynamic process of equilibrium, such as respiration and the sustaining of the major organ's core temperature, are all resolved under the energetic model where all the systems are interdependent.

The outside, back and upper half of the body is classified as Yang, the inside, front and lower half Yin. The meridians or energy channels are coupled in Yin/Yang pairs, liu he.

The heart, lungs, liver, spleen and kidneys are Zhang, full or administrative Yin organs, and correspond to the Five Elements; the Heart's element is Fire, Lungs Metal, Liver Wood, Spleen Earth, and Kidneys Water.

The Fu, empty or receptive Yang organs are the gall bladder, large and small intestines, stomach, bladder and 'Triple Warmer' or San Qiao (a concept of metabolism that has a special function of distributing primal energy to different points of the meridians from the kidney system during prenatal development). Triple Warmer refers to the three chou or levels of the body, the upper respiratory and circulatory system, the middle digestive, and the lower reproductive/eliminative functions.

The Pericardium is another conceptual system that doesn't conform to the Western medical model. Whilst the Triple Warmer transports Qi and is related to the lymphatic system and connective tissue, the Pericardium is a transport medium for the Shen or spirit residing in the heart.

There are two cycles in the Wu Xing; generating and controlling. (Chen and Ko). The generating cycle order is Water, Wood, Fire, Earth, Metal, then back to Water and so on (Water generates Wood which generates Fire etc.). The order of the controlling cycle is Water, Fire, Metal, Wood, Earth, then back to Water and so it continues (Water controls Fire etc.).

The seasons are translated as part of the Wu Xing and have their effects on the body, as do various emotions that are related to each of the Zhang organs. One notion is that each of these organs is 'inhabited' by a ruling spirit. The Heart's Shen has mental, creative properties, the Lungs' Po conducts strength and endurance, the Liver's Hun can generate ESP, the Spleen's Yi is logical and the Kidney's Zhi governs survival drive and will.

Colours are also associated with the organs, and this forms part of a visualisation technique in sending healing energy to afflicted areas.

The twelve meridians and their activity or Qi flow are related to the months and the 365 energy points on the body correspond to the 365 days of the year. Obviously this sort of correspondence is easy to ridicule from an allopathic point of view, but the concept is a metaphorical representation of the individual (microcosm) being unified with the universal (macrocosm). To quote the Hermetic rule, 'As above, so below'.

Prescriptive considerations take into account geography, lifestyle, diet and climate. Many variables for each individual case would be observed. Diagnosis would include noting the patient's complexion and palpating the pulses.

There might be an excess or deficiency in the energy state of any organ. The Yin/Yang balance applies. 'Tonify the deficient, sedate the excess' is a general rule, but it requires a thorough analysis of contributory factors.

The key, according to Huang Ti, to effective health care is the balance of the Yuan Qi. The Yang Sheng Tao, the Way of Cultivating Life, codified a system of healthcare. The Western equivalent was the Hippocratic Corpus, a collection of medical works, most likely by other authors as well as Hippocrates, whose central explanation of health was similarly based on an elemental theory, in this instance the four humours. These body fluids were blood, yellow and black bile, and phlegm, and their qualities of heat, cold, dryness and damp complied with Empedocles' four element theory of the composition of all Matter (Fire, Earth, Air and Water).

As autopsies were forbidden during the Han dynasty this might have influenced the study of more subtle physiological processes and an inward contemplative approach. But certainly the circulatory system was understood and described in the Nei Ching, centuries before William Harvey's discovery of pulmonary circulation.

Just as Western religious sensibility has focused outward, on the personifications of God and Christ, so has medicine seemed to focus on organic studies as fragmentary and divided from the whole. In the West the prevalent view on treatment is specialization. So there are heart specialists, eye specialists, specialists in all manner of individual disease and disorder. Not to say that this is not an effective way of treatment. The film director John Huston, when asked what he attributed his long life to, answered succinctly, 'Surgery'. The Western allopathic medical form has saved countless lives and it can claim the boon of X Rays and the discovery of penicillin. There are however areas where it can go awry.

This is one distinction of Chinese medicine, the assessment and treatment of causes rather than symptoms, where symptoms are seen as signs that the body is trying to restore balance. It doesn't regard these signs as enemies of health to be negated but rather as something to be worked with. A treatment of the person, not the disease.

Another distinctive aspect is the energy model. In Western medical literature the only reference to energy is in the field of psychology, and 'psychic' energy. In China and other Eastern countries it has assumed a very sophisticated level with the correspondence of such principles as the eight-part diagnostic method (hot-cold, interior-exterior, strong-weak, Yin-Yang), Five Element Chen and Ko cycle theory, the meridian system, the hun and p'o or animus/anima concepts and a wealth of other aspects.

Not to get starry-eyed over the 'Mystical East'. It has had its fair share over the centuries of warfare, suppression, poverty, class conflict and downright ignorance, such as the horrific foot-binding practice of the Manchu Dynasty. China was for some time known as 'the sick man of Asia'. A depth of insight into psychological conditions might also be considered as deficient.

But of course every culture has its faults, political and ideological pitfalls. At its best, the Chinese civilization has produced incredible advancements in science and art. It has been said that, to the Chinese, the Industrial Revolution is recent history. Such a statement is not meant in a derogatory way, but rather to illustrate their immense history.

Returning to the individual rather than the generic, I think there is a case to criticize the Western emphasis of external appraisal of the body.

A sense of well-being is not predicated by a perfect state, just as being healthy is not necessarily the same as being fit or vice versa. The supposed norms of physicality are really quite fictional. Typing people is ridiculous, as is realised when taking a look at a crowd; there is no normative case. We are only typed (short, tall, fat, thin) for media ease, because the advertising and fashion worlds and other corporate interests want to create a physical ideal, which is a fiction. Trying to live up to others' artificial ideals is draining, and we do no justice by it to the variety of humanity and our myriad states of being.

Having said that, we still should strive for our own sense of perfection, not to the point of obsession or unhappiness, but because it's natural to seek self-improvement and an optimal existence.

5. BREATHING

'The Breath is the Lord of Strength'. Chinese saying.

Breathing is a unique physiological process in that it can be brought under conscious control as well as being an autonomous function.

THE PHYSIOLOGY OF RESPIRATION

The thoracic cavity consists of the sternum, ribs and intercostal muscles, the 12 thoracic vertebrae and the diaphragm. The lungs fill this space with the heart between. The apex of each lung is a little above the clavicle and the base rests on the diaphragm. The trachea divides into two bronchi, then into bronchioles, alveoli and capillaries. Each lung is surrounded by a membrane, the pleura.

   Rhythmic contraction of the intercostal muscles and diaphragm is caused by impulses from the respiratory centre in the medulla oblongata. There are basically two movements taking place in breathing; inhalation and exhalation. As the diaphragm contracts the chest cavity is enlarged vertically, and from side to side and front to back by the contraction of the intercostal muscles. In exhaling, the relaxation of the muscles forces air out. Oxygen and carbon dioxide are interchanged during the respiratory process. Oxygen, taken in by the nose and mouth, passes int0 the lungs through the alveolar/capillary membrane. It is taken up by haemoglobin in the red blood cells to the heart, and then to all parts of the body. CO_2, as a metabolic waste product, is exhaled.

   At this moment, become aware of your breathing and how you feel as you breathe in, and breathe out. Notice your respiration rate, if it is fast or slow, regular or irregular, deep or shallow. Note if you have tension in any particular area of your body during breathing. Actually feel the air as it comes into and goes out of your body.

The technique of breathing in Qi Gong is called Diaphragmatic or Abdominal breathing. The diaphragm is considered to be the centre of one's strength. The concept is that by focusing attention on the lower half of the torso the breath is deepened and engages the full capacity of the lungs. It's a method that is also used effectively by, for example, opera singers. Sometimes it is described as 'filling the abdomen with breath', which naturally is not anatomically correct but gives a sense of the technique. Simply, as you breathe in, the abdomen expands; upon breathing out it contracts. As a Qi Gong exercise the attention is focused on the navel area, the power centre of the Dan Tien.

Although in most explanations of this method only the forward and backward movement of the abdomen is considered, there is actually a spherical aspect, as the ribcage expands outward laterally, the diaphragm rises and falls and if you place a hand on the area between the kidneys, the Ming Men, as you breathe you will feel a slight movement there too.

Exhalation is a Yang action, as in the primal creative moment, the out breath or 'Word of God'. Inhaling is the Yin withdrawal. Religious or cosmological speculation on the fate of the universe might therefore be phrased in terms of a breathing cycle.

Pranayama, the yogic equivalent of Qi breathing exercises, has a variety of different techniques such as closing one nostril alternately as you breathe, counting up to 4 on the in-breath, 2 on the out-breath, and so on. There is a possibly apocryphal story of a yoga enthusiast who spent so much time engaging in conscious breath control that he lost the autonomic function, and spent an anxious night desperately trying to recover it. True or not there is a little note of caution, a case of Occam's razor. To apply the wisdom of the North, 'If in doubt, do nowt'. Changes in breathing can alter blood chemistry and thus affect cerebral function, as well as incurring other organic conditions.

The method called Rebirthing was developed in the mid-1980s by Leonard Orr. It can be described as 'Conscious Connected Breathing', where there is no pause between the inhalation and exhalation. The idea is that the body's 'cellular memory' (memory that is dispersed throughout the body and not just cerebral) can be activated through this process, releasing past traumas such as birth problems. It has been criticised as being merely over-breathing or hyperventilation, which can cause tetany and panic attacks. Israel Regardie used hyperventilation as part of his clinical work as a psychotherapist, and in 'The Eye in the Triangle' made a comparison between it and pranayama, noticing the similarities in various stages of emotional and physical states (in this respect he could be considered an early Rebirther).

Qi Gong tends towards minimum interference, or making more effective what is natural. The rule is to proceed on the side of caution. Not to say there might not be benefits in exploring the different kinds of breath exercise, but the simplest method seems personally to be as effective, and certainly completely safe.

The channels for increased energy flow must be developed gradually. Just as in developing structural alignment in the body, slow and steady practice is required in order to forge new connectivity.

Embryonic Breathing is very fine, silent breathing, in which a sheet of tissue paper or a feather could be held in front of the nose without being disturbed by the breath. You might find it occurs naturally and incidentally, without being sought, as your concentration deepens during exercise.

One other Taoist technique I will mention, as it is come upon quite frequently in a number of texts especially as relating to Taoist Alchemy, is known as Reversed or Prenatal Breathing. With this method the abdomen contracts as you inhale, and expands as you exhale. It is also used in martial arts, but it is not recommended being used for long periods of time. Essentially, it's a means of stimulating energy.

When Taoist teachers talk about 'whole body' breathing, they are referring to the movement involved throughout the body in respiration, such as how the knees straighten and relax during inhalation and exhalation when practicing standing Qi Gong.

As for combining movement with the breath, such as in the 'active' Qi Gong exercises, then generally the in, Yin, breath is associated with a rising or inward movement; the out, Yang, breath is usually a falling or outward action. For example, the opening of the Yang style Tai Chi form consists of the arms being raised in front of the body until the wrists are at a level approximately with the shoulders; this is on an in-breath. As the arms slowly lower you breathe out. This is also used as a Qi Gong practice in itself, known as the Taoist Water Exercise.

The rate of breathing during Qi exercises is ideally about the same as for the Tai Chi form, around two in and out breaths per minute, but just keep to what is comfortable. Don't force the breath.

Breathing is our constant union with our environment, because we are continually taking in something from what is around us, and giving out the converted energy. The lungs never rest. There is an idea that through the medium of breath one can even institute changes in the surroundings. A personal alchemy.

Qi Gong

Certainly the main prospect in Qi Gong is utilizing breath to enhance the inner state of health and general well-being, quite apart from spiritual considerations.

6. SITTING

'The Way to do is to be' (Lao Tzu).

There are a number of positions and formal postures for seated meditation, such as Seiza or 'correct sitting' in Japan ('sitting meditation' is Zazen). Taoist seated meditation differs from the usual stereotypical seated position of most Eastern meditation in that it doesn't emphasise a lotus or half-lotus posture, and that the soles of the feet are placed flat on the ground. Like kneeling postures, sitting on the ground can prove uncomfortable in Western society, and there has been a study where it has been found that there are actual physiological differences in cultures that are more used to ground-seating than ours, such as a thicker knee joint. Cross-legged positions don't serve to facilitate the movement of energy internally and externally that are the locus of Taoist practices.

The chair-seated position illustrates a general principle in Qi Gong physical alignment of being neither too relaxed to the point where you are liable to fall asleep, nor of holding tension in the body by trying too hard.

The Qi Gong posture in a chair is the middle point between these extremes; relaxed but aligned. The upper legs should be fairly horizontal, parallel with the ground. The back and lower legs are vertical. This position is sometimes known as the Lightning Flash, as it resembles the zig-zag shape generally representative of a bolt of lightning. It is also known as the God or King Posture, based on such images as seated Egyptian statues of pharaohs. The hands are placed on the knees, palms up.

Energetically the position provides a clear channel between Heaven energy coming in through the top of the head and the palms, and Earth energy through the soles of the feet connected to the ground. It ideally accommodates the 'neutral spine', that is, the natural three curves of a healthy spine, the cervical, thoracic and lumbar. The best posture aims to optimize the functions of breathing and circulation.

The great thing about this position is that it can be used for beneficial purpose at any time when you have a spare moment or remember it. Even on a bus or train, or at work. Just taking a few deep breaths will help to still the mind.

Later you will come across a seated meditation that is on the ground, at the end of the Yuan Qi set of exercises, but you will note that this posture entails placing the soles of the feet together to create an energy circuit. The purpose of Taoist seated meditation is primarily containment. We are constantly diverted and lose energy through our senses being distracted, by noise pollution, demands on our time, and the draining effect of our electronic environment. Often people can no longer bear to be alone with their own thoughts but need the security blanket of being plugged into mobile phones, headsets and TV screens, keeping them separated from the real world and also from themselves. In stilling the 'Monkey Mind' that is restlessly caught up in thoughts of past or future, we are simply Being Present. As Jane Roberts in 'The Nature of Personal Reality' put it: 'The point of power is in the present moment'.

The two contrasting forms of meditation are object concentration, where thought is focused upon something, and 'sitting and forgetting', which is more of a free-floating experience of absorption into the Tao. Emptying the mind of thought to achieve a state of emptiness is known as Lien-hsu-ho-Tao, or 'cultivating The Void to merge with the Tao', and is an aim of other traditions as well as a foundation training exercise in some systems of magic. Cultivating quiet helps to regulate emotions.

As The Void, or the Chaotic state of Tao, is the precursor to all things, different traditions all stress the same type of spiritual discipline in getting to a core truth. Tibetan, Gnostic, Chinese, Indian, Sufi, Hebrew and Shamanic esotericism recommends meditation, and in particular motionless cessation of thought (MNT-Motionless No Thought) as an imitative means of returning to The Void in order to penetrate the nature of the external manifest world. Effective meditation, as opposed to mere daydreaming, initiates tangible results. Rather than engaging in such a practice because it is a 'spiritual' thing to do, and ending up enduring it, the only point should be a material product, that is, that it leads to a relatively more healthy, happy and fulfilled existence. Veselin Cajkanovic, the Serbian classical scholar, wrote of sitting as a magical act, 'Magical Sitting', that could connect the individual with other persons or states having occupied that position.

Regarding the psychoanalytic approach, it is not useful to sift through the content of the subconscious, which is sometimes termed meaninglessly 'processing your stuff'. Therein lies madness and the torments of Sisyphus. Far better is to adopt the orientation of the creative. The faculty of visualization has many potent uses, and creative visualization is used to lead or guide energy.

There are guided meditations where imagined scenes that could be happy events or places in one's life, or constructed idealised locations, can provide a peaceful refuge. Initially I just tell people to relax, and let them watch their own thoughts as they flit across their minds, as the first step is keeping the body still, breathing deeply without fidgeting. This alone proves a challenge for some; a fear of silence seems to be equivalent with a fear of the dark. Also, not talking is an exercise in itself. Too much talking dissipates life force; keeping quiet is said to safeguard meridian Qi. Silent sitting is known as Jing-zuo.

The Inner Viewing practice of Nei-shih or Nei-kuan involves visualizing the inside of the body, and is a precursor to such exercises as the 'Inner Smile' where the organs are 'smiled' at (yes, I know it sounds mad, but the principle has a logic; positive energy). This is also coordinated with the use of different coloured energies imagined to be permeating each organ, related to the Five Element theory. As various states of emotional energy are accorded to each organ there is a psychological alchemical aspect of transmuting negative thoughts and feelings. Taoist chants or mantras have further health and consciousness altering attributes. They take the mind out of normal consciousness by the unfamiliar language, promote a sense of 'tuning in' to the current or tradition and, as the science of acoustics relates, have a vibratory effect upon the body.

Subvocal vibration of sound can be utilized if lacking privacy, although this is relatively less potent. The Six Healing Sounds (Liu Zi Jue) is a popular Qi Gong using the intoning of different sounds to resonate with the internal organs (liver, heart, spleen, lungs and kidneys, with the addition of the 'Triple Warmer') or to be more precise, harmonizing with the PRF or Prime Resonant Frequency of each organ. This is not such an unusual concept given the effectiveness of ultrasound treatments as conventional therapy.

The teacher Ni Hua Ching has provided a number of interesting invocations, such as Yi Shi Vi which he corresponds to the three Tan Tien, and he also uses phrases taken from Lao Tzu and Chuang Tzu amongst others.

What you should start to gain through practicing quiet sitting, whether using invocations or not, is a sense of your own internal state, proceeding from feeling the muscles, bones and organs that constitute the physical body. Employing mantras in Taoist meditation is not the same as making 'Affirmations' or 'Positive Thinking'. These do not work (see p.105 of 'The Path of Least Resistance, The Powerlessness of Positive Thinking', for a conclusive refutation). A natural positive attitude is much different from imposing 'positive thoughts' which are not perhaps in accord with your experience of reality.

To make a very fleeting mention of what are known as 'Inner Contacts', there are deities that are traditionally supposed to inhabit the body as well as the Universe. The practice of merging with an image known as 'Assuming a Godform' in Western magical practice, is called 'Visualizing the Valley Spirit' in Taoism. Lao-tzu is a popular choice for this purpose.

As a 'kick-start' to the next phase, either standing or moving exercise, I usually add an An mo meridian points massage to the end of the meditative session. The following three are Lung meridian points. LU1 and LU2 are just under the end of the collar bone, before the bulge of the shoulder. LU5 is on the crease of the elbow outside the biceps tendon.

Points can usually be found as slight depressions (perhaps the reason why they are also referred to as 'cavities') and may feel tender to pressure. Massage using the first and second finger tips, with a rotational action, pushing into the point but without forcing.

Additionally, Ren 17 on the midline at the sternum and midway between the nipples has both an 'opening' and calming effect.

What we have begun to realize with simply sitting is how mental constructs can be potentized by intent, and that the body is amenable to suggestion. Note that we are engaging in sitting practice as a conscious process; sitting for too long in an upright posture can cause stress on the back, and of course numerous medical reports have concluded that a sedentary lifestyle can increase the possibility of developing such conditions as diabetes and heart problems. The best posture for sitting over an extended time, as medically recommended, is to lean back by 45 degrees, with the back naturally supported.

7. STANDING

'Patience is a high virtue'. Chaucer.

The first active physical exercise we engage in is standing. That might seem paradoxical, but there is actually a lot of effort involved in learning how to stand still. It requires an understanding of personal anatomical alignment, respiratory awareness, our own state of relaxation or stress, balance and focus. In fact you soon find that there is a lot of movement involved in keeping still, especially at an internal level. In Qi Gong the mind is more active in a standing position than if lying down or seated

Physiologically, the advantage of our upright posture is that it is easier to carry our relatively large heads upright, providing a better view and transferring weight vertically, which combines with our dexterous hands (freed from the reliance of walking on four limbs like other mammals) to give us a more effective way to use our muscles. 40 per cent of our weight is comprised of skeletal muscle. The disadvantage is that the lower joints of hips, knees and ankles must now bear the weight of the body in transmitting forces to the ground.

Where you stand becomes the central point of your world, the omphalos ('navel', originally a stone artefact used to indicate a central point, as at the Temple of the Delphic Oracle). Trees, towers, ladders and mountains indicate the same connection between heaven and earth (hence the significance of Mt. Fuji in Japan and Kun-Lun in China, as sacred mountains personifying their nations). In its aspect as the embodiment of the Tree of Life the human body is an axis of the world. 'Standing Like a Tree' is a popular description for standing exercises.

To begin with, either an empty stomach or an over-full one can affect your state of mind, so you can have a light snack at least an hour before practice, and leave an hour after exercising before you eat again.

TIME AND ENVIRONMENT

Sunrise is optimally the best time, at least early morning for active energetic exercises as you are then set up for the day. Preferably you can practice outdoors, although it is dependent upon season and climate. Performing Qi Gong standing on grass or earth with bare feet, in natural surroundings such as a park, near a lake or by trees, is ideal. You should be neither too hot nor too cold. Pictures and stories of people practicing in snow or desert are usually of masochistic martial artists, it has to be said. You don't have to suffer (too much) for this art, even though standing in one position for a time requires a degree of steadfastness. Some teachers dictate even the direction you should face; South ideally. I think this instruction may be moderated by circumstance, such as not having the sun in your eyes.

The wind is said to disperse Qi, so also be aware of that, even if working indoors and there's a draught. A tranquil environment is needed. Away from people and traffic noise/pollution, as much as is possible. The idea is not to be distracted, so that also means disconnecting or turning off phones, and just basically setting aside some time for yourself.

CLOTHING

No tight belts, no restriction. A uniform isn't needed but some practitioners find that putting on something like the Tai Chi style outfit helps enhance the effects, getting them in the right frame of mind. I don't recommend the Chinese style slippers with the slippery plastic soles. Light canvas shoes like espadrilles are OK. It's best to remove jewellery and watches, as they can interfere energetically.

STANDING POST (ZHAN ZHUANG)

This basic stance is also known as the Wu Chi stance, Wu Chi being the term for the primordial state of limitlessness, or emptiness.

To start it can be useful to stand in front of a full-length mirror to check your posture. Stand with the feet about shoulder width apart. Imagine that you are standing on parallel lines, and that the outside edge of the big toe and heel of both feet are placed on the lines. Feel where your balance is.

Now adjust your weight back a little onto the heels. At a point a little above the centre of the sole of the foot is Kidney 1, or K1, which is a meridian point. It is also known as the Yong Quan (Bubbling Wells or Bubbling Spring) Point, probably because

Standing

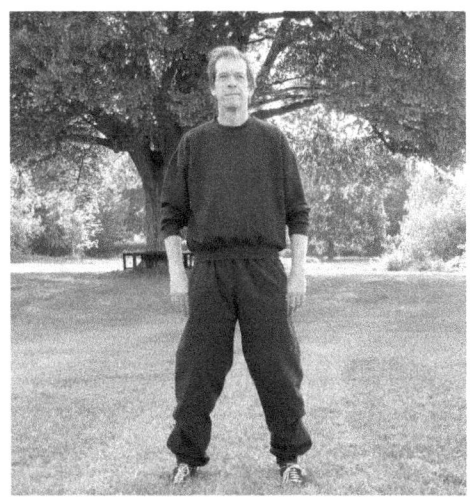

The Wu Chi stance

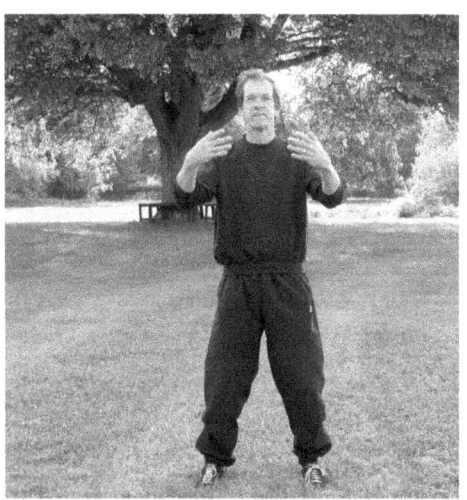

The more advanced posture

of the feeling of earth energy that comes through it. A few Qi Gong teachers advise curling the toes in to raise the sole slightly, but I find that usually creates tension and is hard to maintain initially, so just relax the feet.

Take a breath in and as you exhale sink your weight down, as if you are about to sit down on a chair. The knees should not be pushed forward over the toes. Again, a mirror can help you check this alignment until you are used to the stance.

The coccyx is pointing down, the spine straight. Chuang Tzu said, 'Take your spinal column as your regulating principle'. Obviously, if you look at an anatomical diagram of the spine, it isn't absolutely straight, but has four curves, the cervical, thoracic, lumbar and pelvic, alternately curving forward and backward. But it's easier in this instance to think of the back as simply straight. Tuck your chin in a little and feel the pull upward on the spine as you do so. To borrow from the Alexander Technique, imagine a golden thread attached to the top of your head (the Bai Hui or Du Twenty Point) from which the body is suspended.

Relax the shoulders. Shoulders and neck are particular areas of the body where we can carry a lot of tension because we tend to be upper-body focused.

Relax or 'sink' the chest. You should adopt the opposite effect to the 'soldier on the parade ground' stance in this respect, that is, don't expand the chest.

Let the arms hang at the sides. The inside edges of the hands, the space between the forefinger and thumb where there is a point known as Hegu or LI4, rest on the thighs so the palms face backward. With this arm position the elbows are turned outward so there is space at the axilla (armpit) on both sides.

Either look straight ahead, downward at an angle (still keeping the head straight) or if you find there are visual distractions, close your eyes.

Feel as if your weight is sinking straight down into the ground. The knees should not be bearing weight, they are weight-transference joints. In the spirit of 'Standing like a Tree', imagine there are roots extending from the soles of your feet, just like the roots of a tree, into the ground. This works even if you are indoors and not even on a ground floor, as it is an exercise in imagination, yet it incidentally does affect your sense of balance and 'groundedness'. Feel below the body and above the head.

Unless you have a breathing impediment, the mouth should be closed so you are breathing in and out of the nose. The tip of the tongue is attached to the roof of the mouth, but not too far back; just behind the upper front teeth.

So having checked all these points of alignment, the next step is to relax into it. There is a Chinese term, 'Sung', which translates as something like relaxed awareness. Being alert, not inert. That is the state we are looking for as the body becomes settled into the stance. The body will adjust itself, we don't want to be straining for results. You might have to deal with old patterns of postural habit, so there can be aches and pains at first. Aches are fine; they fade away after continued practice. Specific pain is a warning sign. If that is experienced, stop the exercise and assess the seriousness of the problem.

It is advisable to keep the stance simple at first. There are many other forms of Standing Post that involve holding the arms in different positions, but as these tend to increase tension they are best left to a later stage when the practitioner has had some practice in remaining still for a fair amount of time. Also, holding the arms up distracts from integrating the various fundamental elements of the stance.

As you are standing you will find the legs beginning to shake. This occurs even if you have strong leg muscles, because we are not using muscular strength in the exercise but form integration. Just breathe and keep relaxing. The tremors stop after a while or may change to a mild and not unpleasant 'buzzing' sensation. Of course if the shaking does not stop then do not carry on. You do not want to try too hard with the practice, it's not a case of 'no pain, no gain'. Just as in Tai Chi, once you get the legs right, everything else follows.

You might try a step by step method of relaxing each part of the body from the top of the head to the toes. Feel the difference when you tense the muscles of the forehead by frowning; you can feel the tension right up to the top of the head. Now release the frown, in combination with an out breath. You can work down the rest of the body in this manner, out through the arms to the fingertips, down through the trunk and down the legs to the toes. Or you can imagine your attention as a transverse plane of light slowly descending from the crown of the head to the feet and melting away areas of tension.

Slowly build up the amount of time you stand for. Everyone varies as to how much time will be of benefit. Even just taking five minutes to de-stress can be helpful. Gradually work up by increments to half an hour and take it from there. At the extreme end of the scale are martial artists using standing post in its function as the fundamental power training method of the Chinese internal style martial arts, and who can maintain a stance for an hour, or even hours. There is a point of diminishing returns at that level. In standing over an extended period of time in a session, tension creeps in, and you'll suddenly become aware of such things as your shoulders having almost imperceptibly lifted up. Release the tension by dropping it downward with an out breath. Release in standing is always downward, into the ground.

In the more advanced raised arm postures, stress is felt in the shoulders, and the lung points at the front of the body between shoulders and chest can particularly feel tense. Also the upper back and neck. If you feel heat rising into the head, breathe or blow out through the mouth a few times to dispel it. Naturally you should stop if the experience persists.

After a while you find the greatest problem to overcome is your own mind. As classic texts such as the Dhammapada relate, the mind is the enemy. It must be destroyed! Well, certainly tamed.

You will find excuses coming up for not practising, distractions, boredom. Watch your thoughts float by like clouds and allow them to pass. Keep committed. The only way to gain positive results is through consistency.

Music can be useful in the background, particularly as an aid in time-keeping because you don't want to be continuously clock-watching. If you know how long a piece is then you won't be continually distracted by thoughts of what the time is, how long you've held the stance and how much longer you have. Heavy metal at full blast is not recommended.

CONCLUSION

At the end of your session, slowly raise your arms out to the sides, as if they are being drawn upward by threads attached to your wrists, and at the same time take a deep breath in.

The hands float in until the fingertips are opposite each other but not touching and just level with the Mid-brow Point. Pause for a moment, and then with a slow exhalation bring the hands down the front of the body until they are level with the Dan Tien. Fold the hands over this area, men hold the right hand over the left, women the left hand over right, and relax. Position of the hands is related to Yin/Yang balance.

Placing the hands over the Dan Tien 'stores' the Qi.

Take a few breaths, then slowly start to come out of the stance. Rock back and forth a little on your feet, step up and down, give your arms a gentle shake, and begin to move around, adjusting back into movement.

The awareness in standing goes through stages, from concentration on muscles and joints, to the internal organs, and after a while to feelings around and outside of the body, so what you can feel is like a bubble of energy around you, which is known through various esoteric traditions as the aura.

The natural order is to go from a conscious awareness of energetic inner states to the external environmental energy, and then to a sense of others as energetic beings. The circle around ourselves includes and excludes, just as through our breathing we take in and give out.

Sometimes I have found people have a sense of falling even though they are standing still. Balance leans upon gravity, and the fear of falling is a fundamental one; being 'brought down to earth', like the shock fall that wakes us at times from dreams (there is a view that this is due to our leaving our physical bodies when in the dream state, then 'falling back' into them when we awake, especially if woken suddenly).

The Fall is a vital, archetypal symbol, and it is useful to reflect on its effects. In a Hapkido class when I was thrown a few times and landed painfully, I was taught that if we 'receive' the ground we can lessen the impact. Another example is falling on icy ground; there is a split-second point at which you realise you are falling, and it then benefits you to go with the fall, as it will therefore have less impact than resisting it. 'Resistance is futile', at least in this instance.

If you feel off-balance in the stance, try bringing your weight backward and forward until you feel a central connection, as you sink down into the ground. Project your mind under your feet. The centre of the body and the central line of the spine grow out of the ground. We are creatures of the earth; this is our natural environment. And we are also between heaven, or the sky, and earth. It is interesting how we might lack that spatial awareness.

A simple exercise for gaining an immediate sensation of Qi is to bounce up and down on the balls of the feet, heels off the ground and not making contact with it as you bounce. Continue for a few minutes then stop, standing still and feeling the 'buzzing' effect through the body.

If practicing standing post for a long session then it is helpful to include a warm-up/cool-down set at the beginning and end, consisting of swinging or gently shaking the arms and legs. Arm swinging is a Qi Gong in itself.

8. THE MERIDIAN ENERGY MODEL

The twelve main meridians in Chinese traditional medicine are each named for an association with a particular organ. For example, the Heart meridian, or Lung meridian.

Points located on the meridians are numbered thus for example; H1 for Heart meridian point 1, or L14, Lung meridian point 14. The eight extra meridians, the Chi-jing ba-mai, are referred to variously as Channels, or even Psychic Channels, Vessels or Reservoirs to differentiate them from the organ meridians. Homeostatic, Ancestral and Miraculous are other prefixes sometimes used, indicating the different aspects of their importance.

These act as storage mediums for Qi, and provide one of the main frameworks for Qi Gong practice. They consist of the Ren Mo or Conceptual Vessel which runs in a straight line down the front of the body from the lower lip to the perineum, the Du Mo or Governing Vessel which runs from there up the back, over the top of the head and down to the upper palate, the Chong Mo or Thrusting Channel that runs through the centre of the body from base of trunk to top of head, the Dai Mo, Belt or Girdle Channel that encircles the waist, the Yin and Yang Qiao Vessels (Qiao means heel, a reference to the promotion of mobility), and the Yin and Yang Wei or Protective Vessels, connecting the meridians together and promoting balance.

The luo, collateral meridians, connect with the 365 points of the system, and are involved with the flow of nutritional and defensive Qi.

ENERGY POINTS ON THE REN AND DU CHANNELS.

The Yin Tang point between the eyebrows is known as the upper Dan Tien, the

Heavenly Pool or palate. By placing the tip of the tongue, which relates to the heart in TCM, to the roof of the mouth, the Ren and Du channels are connected in a circuit. Ren 17, in the midline between the nipples, can be massaged to release stress and emotional blocks or withheld feelings.

The middle Dan Tien relates to the solar plexus area. The lower Dan Tien is about three finger widths below the navel, and can be thought of as a Qi storage area. The Sexual Centre is known by the delightful names of the Sperm Palace or (obviously in the case of women) the Ovarian Palace.

The Perineum, Hui-Yin, is called The Gate of Life and Death. The point beyond it, GV1, brings energies up the spinal column. The Sacrum is known as the Immortal Bone, possibly due to its eight holes.

The Ming-Men, between the kidneys, translates as The Door of Life. The left kidney is Yin, the right Yang, and they represent mother and father.

The centre opposite the heart, T11, is an area of 'hot' energy.

C7, the large vertebra opposite the throat, is a junction for nerves of the hands and legs.

At the base of the skull, the Jade Pillow or God Mouth has a role in breath regulation and the promotion of Yin energy.

The Bai Hui or Meeting Place of a Thousand Spirits at the top of the head is in Taoist alchemical practice related to the North Pole and cosmologically to the North Star. It 'opens' to receive Heavenly Qi. Also it connects to the Pineal gland and mid-brain in the reception of knowledge.

9. OCCULT ANATOMY

'I Sing the Body Electric'. Walt Whitman.

I first came across the term Occult Anatomy in J.H. Brennan's 'Experimental Magic'. The idea is of a science of supra-physical structure outside the realm of common biological explication.

Various cultures have traditions of a subtle energetic physiology, some of their features being practically identical. The following is a basic enumeration of just a few of the correspondent attributions and is by no means exhaustive. The meridian model can as example be added.

The Ying Tang or 'Third Eye' point is represented in the wearing of the bindi by women throughout South Asia (Chinese women used to wear marks on their foreheads during the Tang Dynasty, but possibly only for decorative reasons). It is known as one of the Chakras (Sanskrit for Wheel) in the Indian concept of esoteric anatomy, is concerned with intuition and psychic perception, and named Ajna. Associated with the pituitary and pineal glands, it is considered a vestigial remnant of the reptilian brain. Such mythic creatures as the Unicorn and Cyclops might be taken as symbolic of the third eye, and it may be referenced in the Bible, Matthew 6:22; 'The lamp of the body is the eye: if therefore thine eye be single, thy whole body shall be full of light'. Other references to it include the descriptions 'the central white light' and 'the light of the sacred square inch' between the eyes, in the Taoist canon.

The Throat area is known as Heaven's Projection in Taoist Qi Gong and is associated with the practice of 'Dream Yoga' or work undertaken on the Astral Plane. Conscious dreaming, becoming aware during a dream, is a method of training in certain occult schools. Dreams can represent aspects of the self that are 'unexpressed', a corollary of which is the Taoist idea that if you are fully at ease within yourself you don't dream.

As the Visuddha Chakra, it relates to communication and sound vibration. The voice can be used for healing, as with prayer, recitation, singing and so forth, or as a weapon to inflict psychic harm; not necessarily so obviously as a blatant curse, but in our daily relations with others. It might be a consciously chosen word or how someone takes a remark personally that could have been made in all innocence, 'seeding' a word into a person's psyche, a little like the subliminal messages used in advertising. This is the location of the Qabalistic Sephira Daath, a junction dividing thought (the head) from feeling (the body).

There is a proposal in some occult writings that the head occupies a different time frame from the rest of the body. What the ramifications of this may be are anyone's guess.

The Heart or Anahata Chakra is the centre of love and self-acceptance. It is also symbolized by the element of Air. Tiphareth, Beauty or Harmony, is the Sephira located here.

The solar plexus is said to control the aura and act as a meeting point for spiritual energy. It is a very important nerve centre and reacts to stress, as with the 'butterflies in the stomach' sensation. It is advised as a magical defence technique to protect oneself by visualising a shield of some description covering this point. The Manipura Chakra's province at this area is in terms of Ego identity, Energy and Will. Its element is Fire.

The Svadhisthana or Sacral Chakra located in the pelvic area governs emotions and sensuality and relates to the Water element, although in Tibetan Buddhism it is the Fire centre. Yesod is the Sephira titled 'Foundation'.

The Kundalini experience of sexual, earth force arises from the Muladhara, Base Chakra which defines our survival instincts and sheer physicality. The element Earth is therefore symbolized here. Kundalini is the Shakti, 'feminine' energy that rises up the spine to unite with the 'masculine' polarity of the Crown centre. Some societies such as the Freemasons and the OTO organize their levels of initiation on the principle of the 'Spirit Fire' rising through the 33 vertebrae of the spinal column, with 33 degrees (apart from the serpent, the scorpion with its stinging tail, is another symbol of the 'spinal fire', with Scorpio being a sign of occult initiation).

The Dan Tien are controlled by 'gates' that energetically relate to the spine - the lower Dan Tien is at the Ming Men point, storing and transmuting generative energy into vital energy. The middle relates to the Du 14 point between the shoulder blades and changes vital Qi into spiritual Qi. The upper point's gate is the Jade Pillow, where the spine enters the skull. This elixir field functions to merge the spirit Qi with the primordial essence of Tao.

The Sahasrara or Crown Chakra, is a point that can access an influx of spiritual inspiration and guidance, universal consciousness, feelings of the oceanic and holistic, as represented by Kether in the Qabalistic Tree.

Eric Steven Yudelove, in his excellent book 'The Tao and the Tree of Life' (p.109), remarks on the similarity of the Taoist and Qabalistic systems by noticing that the number of Paths on the Tree (32) is the same as the number of major meridians (12 paired organ related meridians and 8 psychic channels).

Spiritual energy flow emphasis, such as the Kundalini effect, can be deleterious if the body hasn't been properly prepared for it. The sort of psychic phenomena that can be experienced at this point are generally warned about as phases rather than ends in themselves. It is always important to have access to a reliable instructor and avoid the practice of uni-directional energy flow, thinking instead of it as akin to working with electricity; the necessity of grounding the current and the use of a circuit.

Naturally people with deep-seated mental/emotional issues should not be practicing the opening of psychic channels of perception In effect, everyone undertaking such work should be using safeguards. Energy in this context is not merely a psycho-physiological process but manifests on a very subtle level that can't be intellectualised; it needs to be intuited.

THE AURA

The aura is another aspect of the 'subtle body' that is represented in various cultures and in different schools of occult thought. There is naturally the sceptic's contention that seeing an aura is the result of visual disturbance, the use of psychotropic drugs or other mundane reasons.

The aura is significant in bioenergetics and energy medicine as a method of diagnosis, and there are a number of levels and colours attributed to it which can represent aspects of emotional and intellectual health or disorder, as well as organic conditions. Bohm's idea of an interpenetrative field effect is perhaps comparable to the Chinese concept of Shen as a spiritual energy field.

Continuous ritual practice such as daily use of a Banishing Ritual is credited with manifesting a 'tangible' aura, and the same effect is associated with Tai Chi and Taoist masters, as if they can create a Star Trek type force field around themselves. Particular development of prenatal energy in Qi Gong is said to confer the ability to see auras.

The images of haloes around the heads of saints and other devout figures, and angels' wings, might also be connected to the concept of the aura.

The chakras are a part of this auric field, as well as being attached to the central channel, the Sushumna, and interacting with the endocrine and lymphatic systems. There is a particular relationship with the pineal, pituitary and thymus glands and the crown of the head, brow and heart.

The necessary point of working with these various components of subtle anatomy is to actually feel them, rather than simply imagining them.

On occasion spontaneous realizations of energy occur, and in fact I have had people telling me of feeling such effects as 'a tingling sensation' up the spine after or during a basic Qi Gong class without knowing beforehand any details of these concepts or my having directed them in such practice. The other area that seems to uniquely 'open' in many people with no previous training or consideration is the top of the head. This is in any case a sensitive area if we think of the fontanel as being open at birth.

Thus far for theory. The allocation of purpose and value are the areas of contention. As to the physiological bases for these collective constructs, in terms of the nervous, lymphatic, glandular and circulatory systems and their vital areas we can see it is quite apparent localized sensations arise due to signal effects of network foci, so there is some validation in an empirical source. Additionally these templates fulfil a particular need, and act collectively as aggregates of coherent experience in spiritual questing. They could be accorded in that manner the status of myth, defining myth as a vital current force of psychic integration.

As Mary Caine wrote that 'Myth illumines and makes sense of history', perhaps it can do the same for biology. An entire story then unfolds that might be titled 'Biomyth', complementing the chapter to follow on the Geomythic.

10. THE EIGHT TRIGRAMS AND THEIR CORRESPONDENCES

		ENERGY BODY	QUALITY	MERIDIAN
Chi'en	Heaven	Physical	Creative	Du
K'un	Earth	Qi	Receptive	Ren
Li	Fire	Psychic	Spiralling & Coiling	Dai
Kan	Water	Causal	Wave Energy	Yang Wei
Sun	Wind	Emotional	Amorphous	Yin Wei
Ken	Mountain	Individuality	Stillness & Light	Yin Chiao
Chen	Thunder	Thinking	Sudden Shock	Chong
Tui	Lake/Cloud	Tao	Formlessness	Yang Chiao

	ANIMAL FORMS	BODY AREAS
Chi'en	Lion	Head
K'un	Unicorn	Stomach, Legs
Li	Hawk	Chest, Heart
Kan	Snake	Abdomen, Kidneys
Sun	Phoenix	Large Intestine, Feet
Ken	Bear	Back
Chen	Dragon	Hips, Liver
Tui	Monkey	Shoulders, Lungs

THE FIVE ELEMENTS CORRESPONDENCE

ELEMENT	ORGAN	SEASON	COLOUR
Wood	Liver/Gall Bladder	Spring	Green
Fire	Heart/Small Intestine	Summer	Red
Earth	Stomach/Spleen	Late Summer	Yellow
Metal	Lungs/Large Intestine	Autumn	White
Water	Kidneys/Bladder	Winter	Black/Blue

The Eight Trigrams and their Correspondences

ELEMENT	EMOTIONS (YANG/YIN)	SENSES	DIRECTION
Wood	Anger/Kindness	Eyes	East
Fire	Hate/Joy	Tongue	South
Earth	Worry/Openness	Mouth	Middle
Metal	Sadness/Courage	Nose	West
Water	Fear/Gentleness	Ears	North

When practicing walking exercises, stepping can be correlated to the Five Element model and affect the corresponding energy system:

Wood	Retreat
Fire	Step Right
Earth	Central Equilibrium
Metal	Advance
Water	Step Left

TIMES OF PEAK ENERGY FLOW THROUGH THE MERIDIANS

Lung: — 3-5 am

Large Intestine: — 5-7 am

Stomach: — 7-9 am

Spleen: — 9-11 am

Heart: — 11 am -1pm

Small Intestine: — 1-3 pm

Bladder: — 3-5 pm

Kidney: — 5-7 pm

Pericardium: — 7-9 pm

Sanjiao: — 9-11 pm

Gall Bladder: — 11 pm -1 am

Liver: — 1-3 am

The optimum time for Qi Gong practice would be during the lung meridian's peak flow, three to five in the morning. Good luck with that! Personally I'm still asleep then.

There was a report a few years ago on the high incidence of heart attacks occurring during midday. Whether that has a correlation with the heart meridian peak flow is a case for speculation.

THE CIRCULATORY FLOW OF QI

Earth to Heaven Yin Energy — flows up the front of the legs and down the outside of the arms, and up the spine.

Heaven to Earth Yang Energy — flows down the front of the body, up the inside of the arms and down the backs of the legs.

THE YUAN QI EXERCISES - Primordial Energy

The following exercises are a direct lineage transmission from Mt. Emei, Szechuan Province. Also known as Emei Shan and Mt. Omei, it is a sacred mountain; formerly a Taoist retreat, most of its temples were converted to Buddhism from the 3rd century AD onward. It is particularly renowned as a centre of Baguazhang practice.

On a cosmic scale, primordial energy can be compared with dark energy, a hypothetical form permeating the universe. At a smaller level it constitutes the human biofield.

The exercises are performed in order as a set, three times each one. They are also known as the Prenatal Energy exercises, or for short, the Prenatals. I was advertising classes at one time using that description, but as a number of pregnant ladies began turning up with an obviously mistaken idea about it, I now use the term 'Yuan Qi exercises' to avoid confusion. Other than in the case of pregnancy and during the period, these exercises can be used by both women and men.

Numbers in brackets refer to photo illustrations.

No.1

THE OPENING EXERCISE

First, adopt the Wu Chi Stance. Take a slow breath in, then out, calming the mind. You may if you wish recite a short mantra, 'I am Air. I am Light. I am Water', imagining yourself as you take a breath in and out for all three transforming into each element.

Now raise the hands slowly until they are at about navel level, palms facing one another, as if you are holding a ball.

Qi Gong

Thumbs lightly extended so there is a space at the 'Dragon's Mouth', the area between the bases of thumb and forefinger. The hands are at such a distance from the body that the imagined ball merges slightly into the stomach area. (1)

Smile! Smiling 'switches on' the meridians.

Bring your arms straight out to the sides, palms upward around shoulder level, without tension. Do not straighten the elbows.

Simultaneously tilt the head gently back so you are looking straight up, pushing the pelvic area forward as you stand on the edges of the feet and taking a deep breath in. (2)

Feel or imagine energy coming into the Ying Tang or third eye point. The Lao Gong points in the palms should also feel activated.

The Yong Quan points on the soles of the feet are meanwhile disconnected from the ground.

The point Ren 17 is opened in this posture, and the Conceptual Vessel activated.

At the end of the in-breath, slowly start to 'close in' your body; the feet are placed flat again, knees come together, arms come in and backs of the hands are joined together below the knees as you bend forward with the out-breath.

Again all these movements are performed simultaneously. (3, 4)

This posture opens Du 14 and the Governing Channel.

At the end of the exhalation, slowly straighten back up with an inhalation, then breath out and relax.

Turn the palms to face down to connect with Earth energy. (5, 6)

My teacher compared this exercise to 'Opening and closing like a flower'. As a gentle spinal stretch method it stimulates the flow of cerebrospinal fluid.

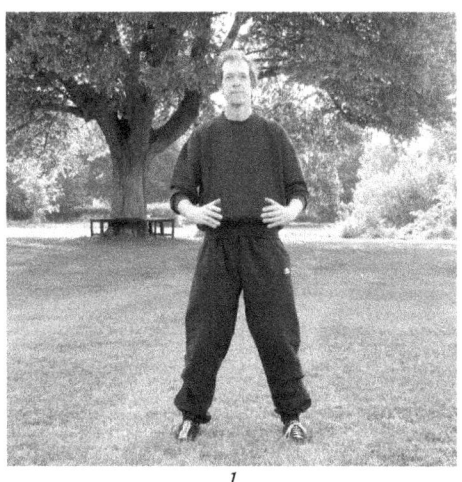

1

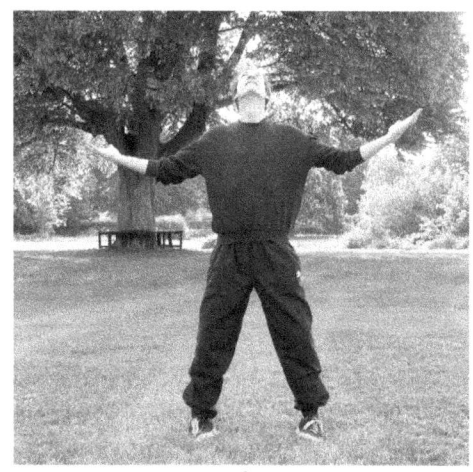

2

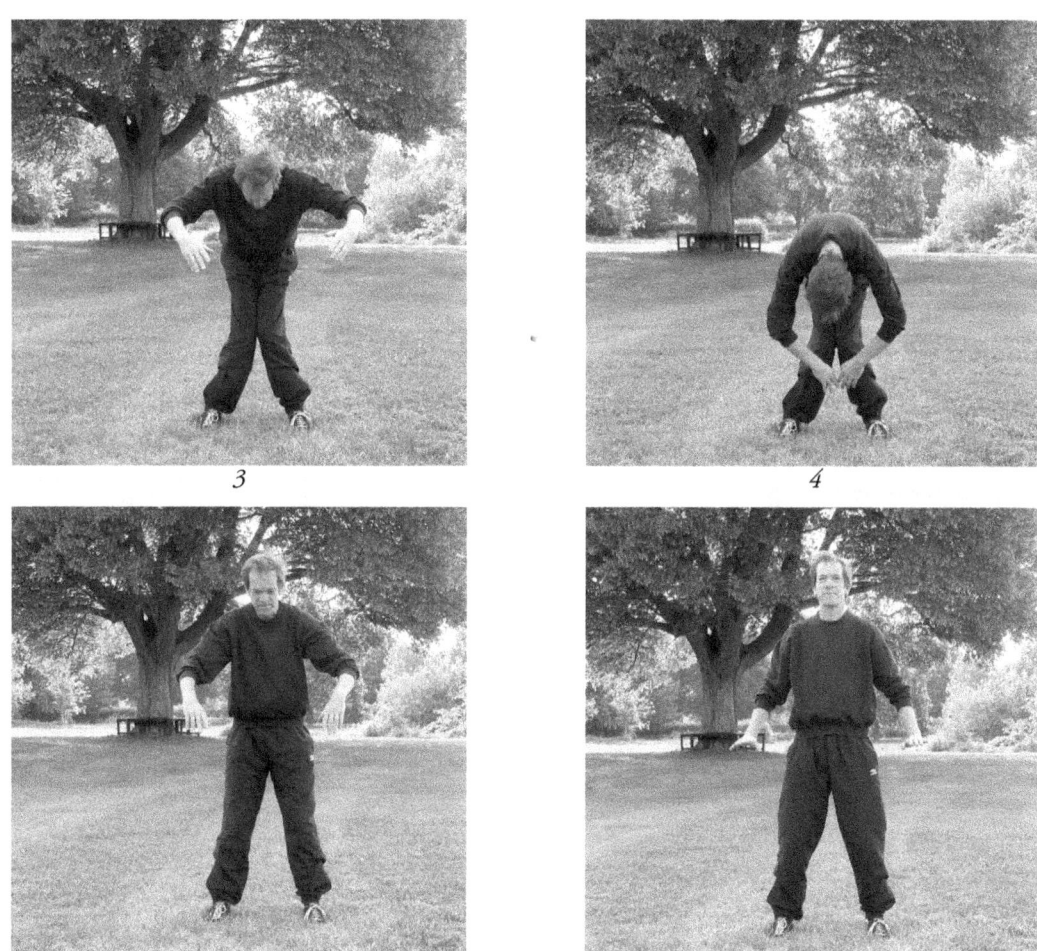

No.2

THE SMALL CIRCULATION OF QI

From the initial posture, holding the ball, hands to waist and step out with the left foot to a 45 degree angle. Shift the weight onto it, hands moving forward and imagine energy flowing down the front Ren Channel from the Dan Tien to the Hui Yin point (perineum). Sink slightly down with the out-breath. (1, 2, 3)

Bring the hands back to about hip level, palms facing backward, as you shift the weight back to the right foot. Imagine energy flowing up the Du Channel from the Hui Yin very slowly with the in-breath, vertebra by vertebra. (4)

When it reaches the back of the neck, at the C7 point, gently lift the head to look up. Feel energy flowing over the back of the head and past the Crown, the Bai Hui, until it reaches the Third Eye.

Then tilt the head to look down, bringing the hands forward into the Holding the Ball position, as you breath out visualizing energy flowing down the front of the body to the Dan Tien again. (5, 6)

Bring the left foot back, slowly lift the head to look forward, arms gently fall with palms turned down, breathing in then slowly out, relax. (7, 8)

Repeat on the right side.

The Small Circulation has also been called The Water Wheel, a description stemming from the usual fondness of the ancient Taoists for using imagery associated with water.

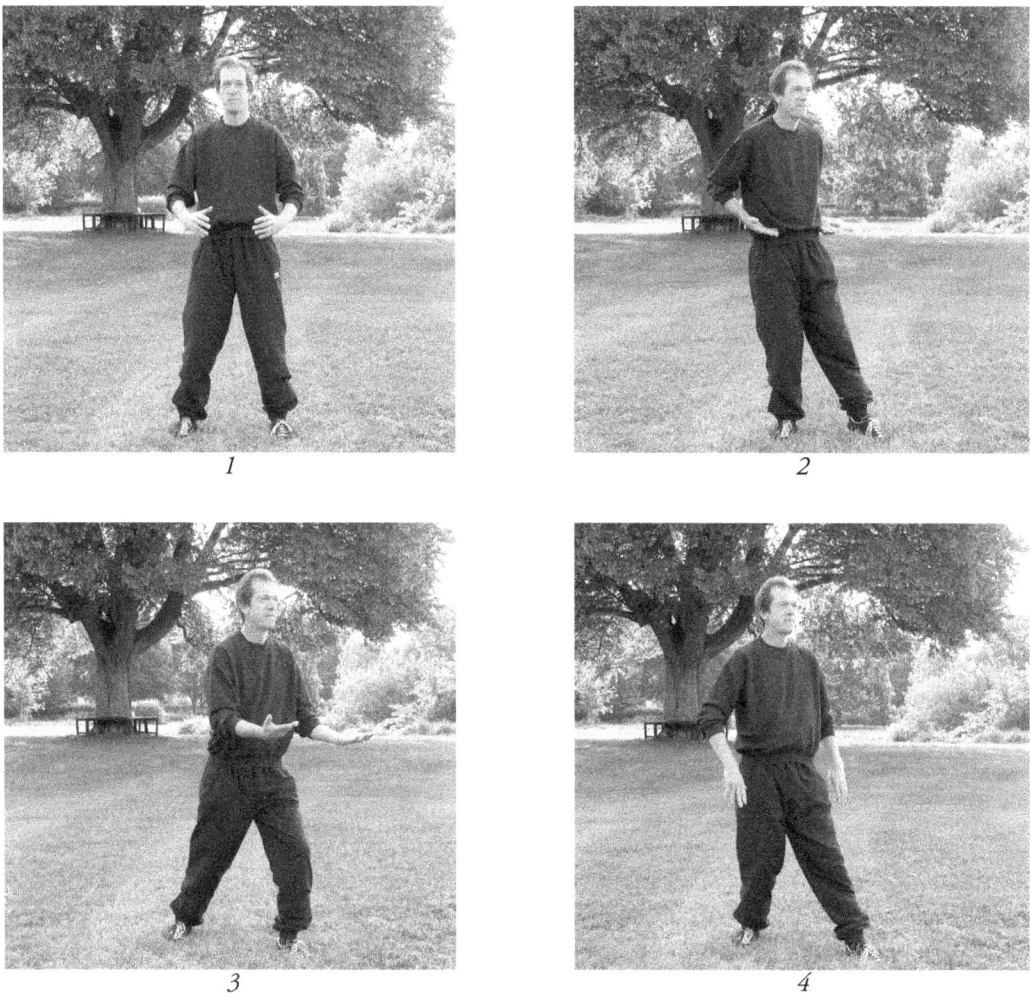

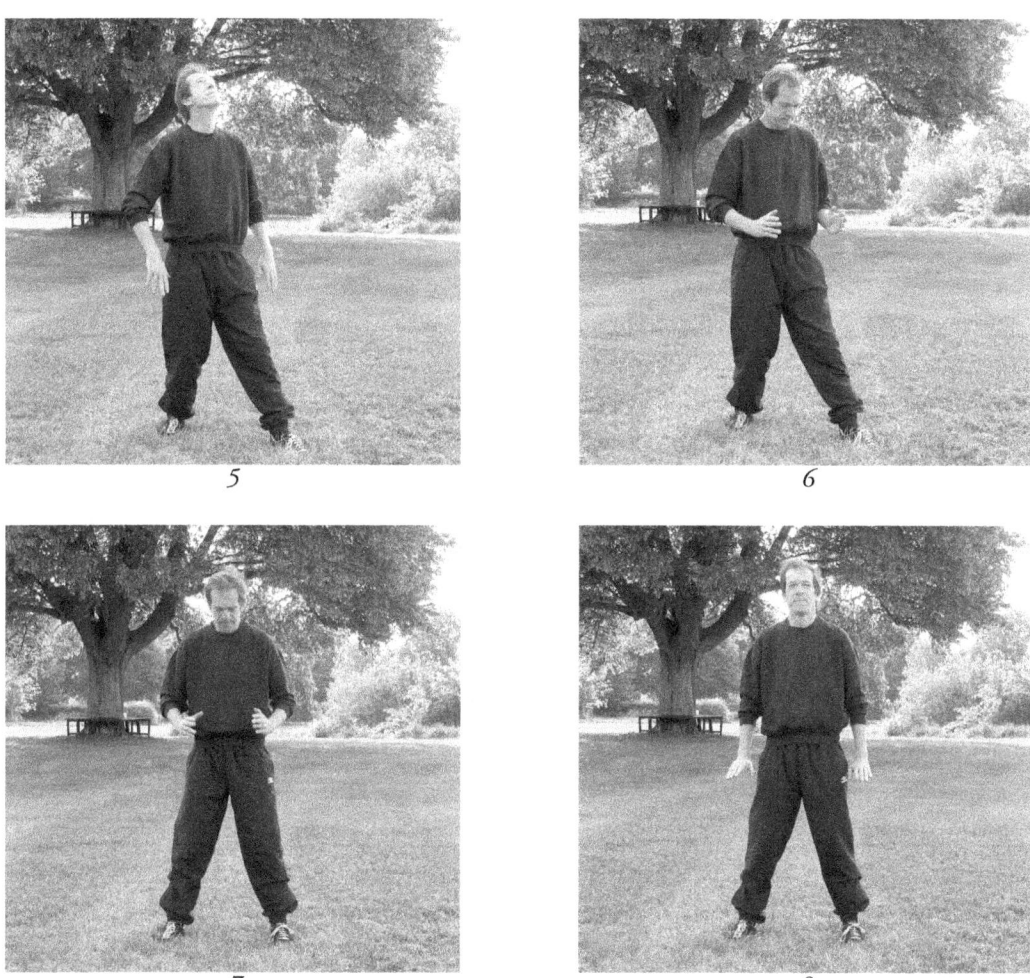

No.3

THE THRUSTING CHANNEL

From the preparatory stance, breathe out as you drop the hands down until the fingertips meet, and then start to curl them inward so the backs of the fingers come together, fingers pointing up. At the same time begin breathing in. (1, 2, 3)

As the hands rise up the centreline of the body the backs will continue to be brought together, until the fingertips are underneath the jaw. As you reach the end of the inhalation pause and feel the heat/energy emanating from the ends of the fingers. (4)

Now upon exhalation the backs of the hands start to rotate outward as the palms are raised in front of the face. The edges of the hands are kept together as you look into the palms. (5)

Feel the heat from the Laogong points entering the eyes. Breathing in, separate the hands out and turn them to an oblique angle upward. Incline backward slightly and tilt the head to look up. Connect with Heavenly Qi through the Laogong and Third Eye Points. (6, 7, 8)

Breathing out, the body straightens and the movements are reversed, the hands coming back together in front of the face with edges connected, looking at the Laogong Points. Backs of hands together, fingertips under the chin breathing in, then continuing the movement down the front of the body as you exhale. (9, 10, 11, 12)

Fingers pointing down, separate the hands and flex the wrists so the palms connect with Earth energy once again. Relax. (13, 14)

Known as the 'Mirror' exercise because of looking into the hands, a movement in common with a Sufi Circle Dance I observed.

The dance forms of different traditions often have an esoteric aspect; for example Flamenco moves portray martial intent.

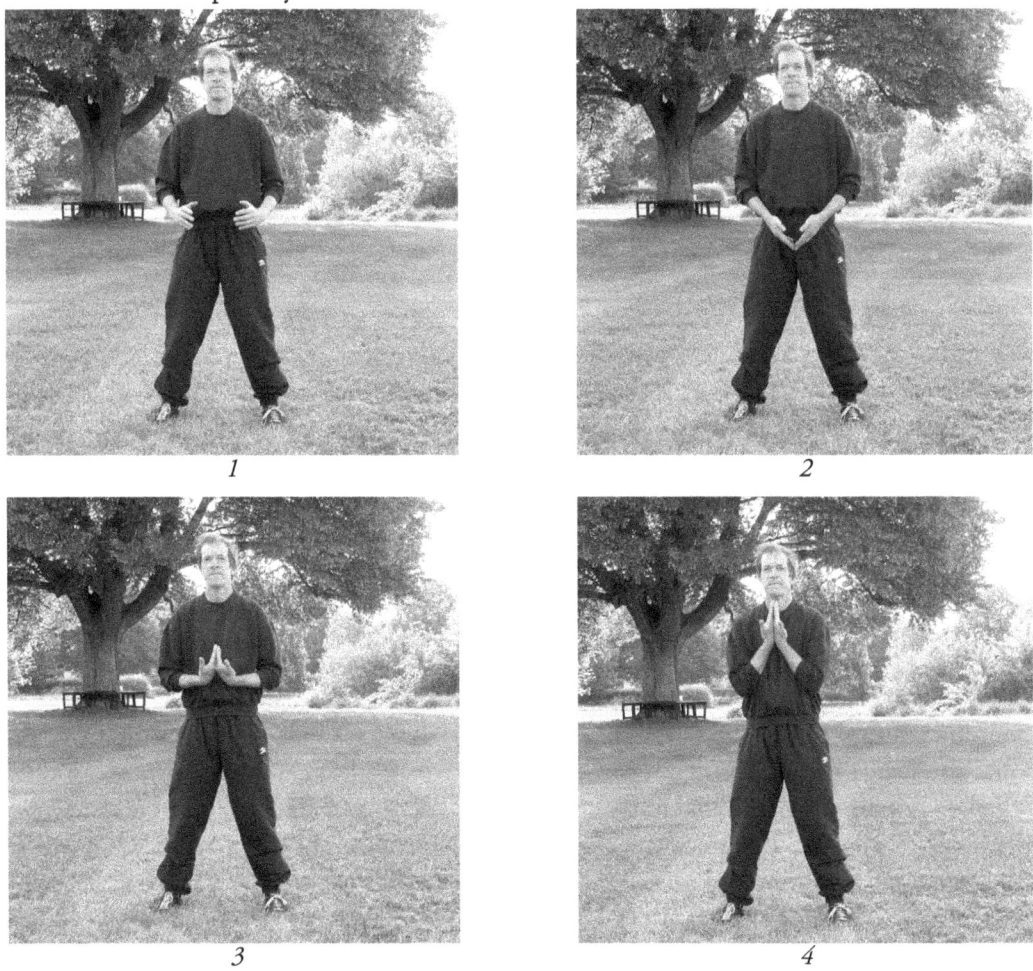

1

2

3

4

The Yuan Qi Exercises

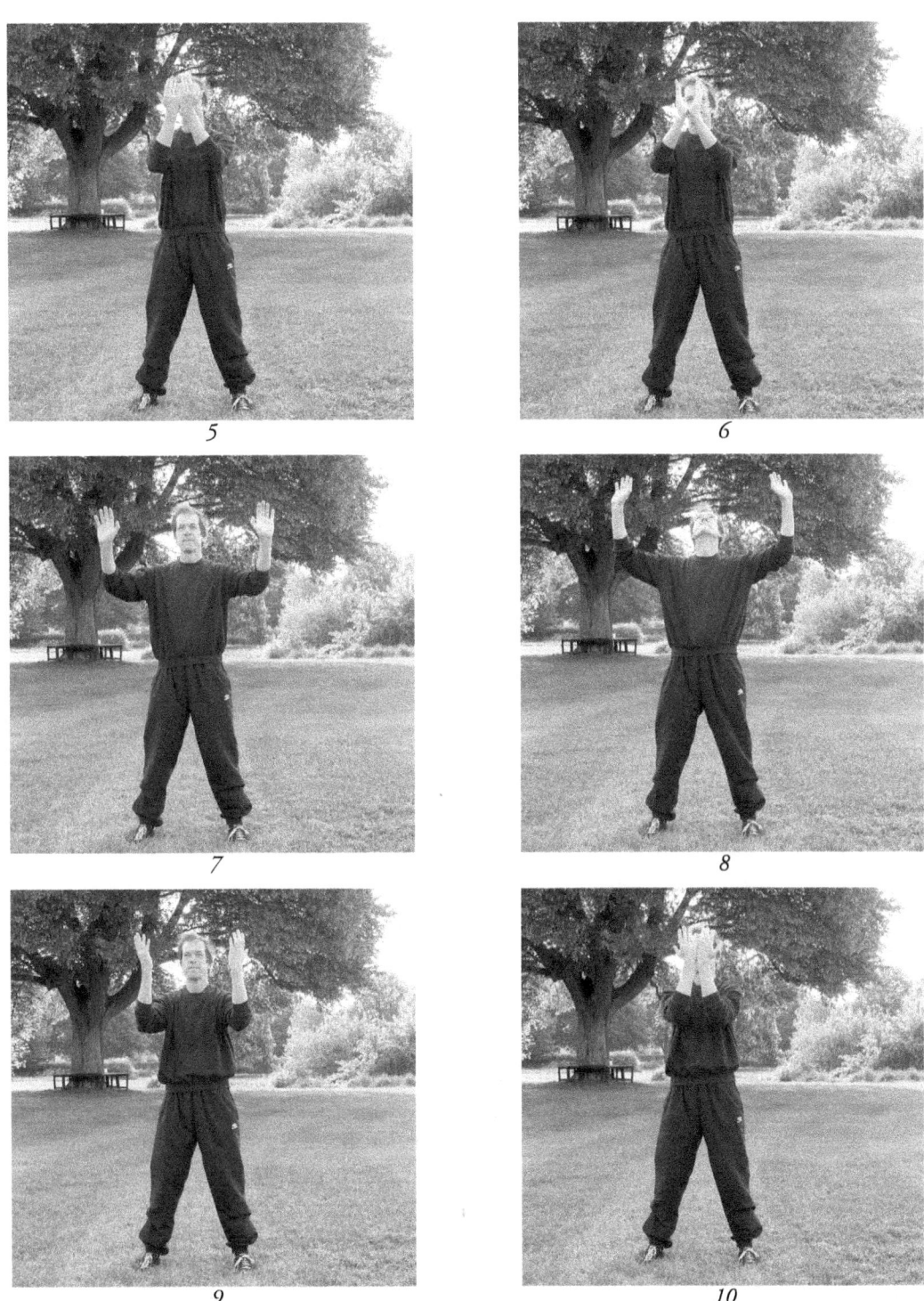

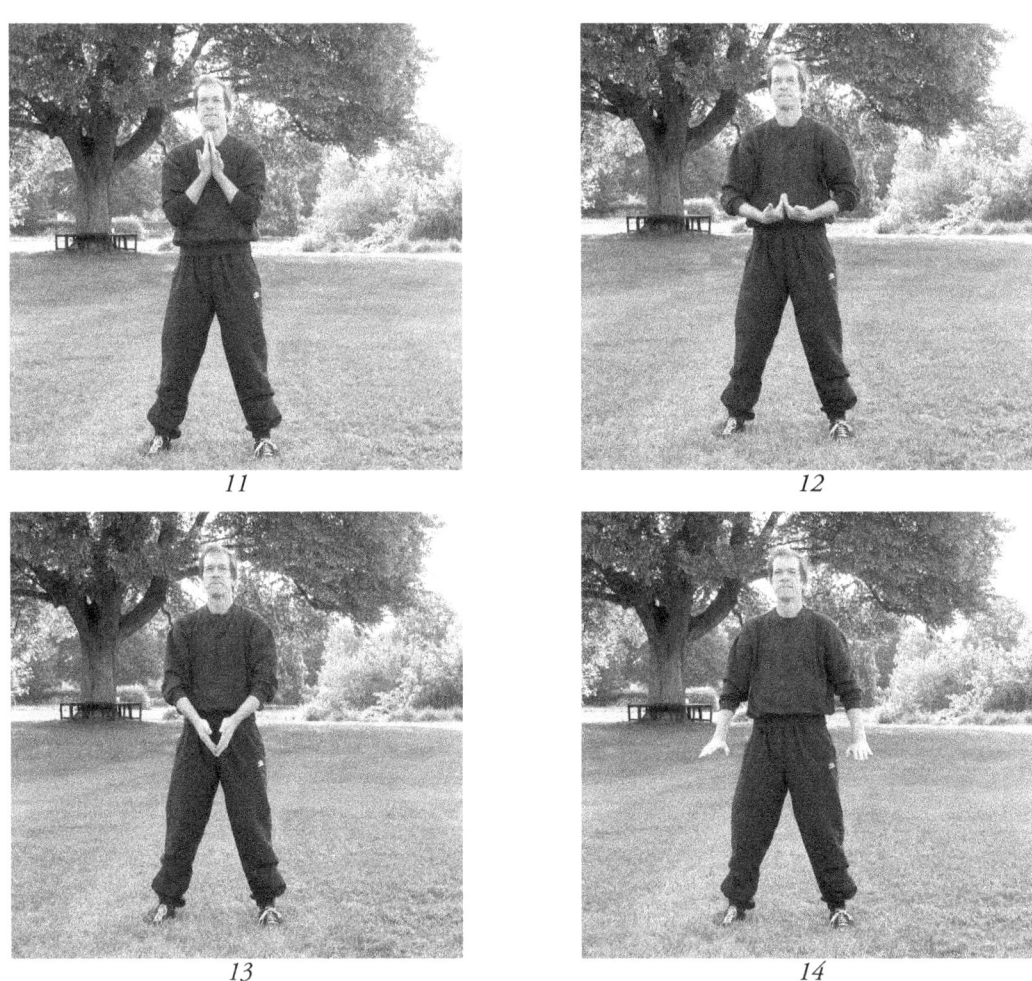

No.4

ARM MERIDIANS

From the Holding the Ball position, the hands fold inward, edges resting on the Dan Tien, back of the left hand lying in the right palm. (1, 2)

With an inhalation, bring the right hand out and above the left, then exhale and press the back of it down into the left palm. (3, 4)

Inhaling, turn the upper body to the left as the left hand is brought around the side, fingers pointing in. Connect the Large Intestine 4 Point (the Dragon's Mouth) with the Ming Men (Du 4), looking behind. (5)

Turn to face forward, breathing out, and simultaneously bring the left hand forward and upward, fingers pointing up. (6, 7)

The Laogong Point is now in front of the Third Eye Point. Pause, breathing normally,

The Yuan Qi Exercises

as you establish a connection between the two centres. You can bring the hand in and out until you get a feeling of warmth between the two points.

Inhaling, turn the waist to the right, then to the left with the hand still held in place. (8, 9)

Lift the elbow, as if the arm is on a pivot, so the fingers are now pointing to the right. Turn to face the front again. (10, 11)

Slowly lower the hand down the front line of the body as you breathe out. (12)

Press the back of the hand into the right palm, which has remained in position throughout the exercise. (13)

Relax and repeat on the other side.

This exercise affects the meridians through the rotational movement. Moving Qi to the ends of the fingers and toes stimulates the corresponding organs according to the meridian system.

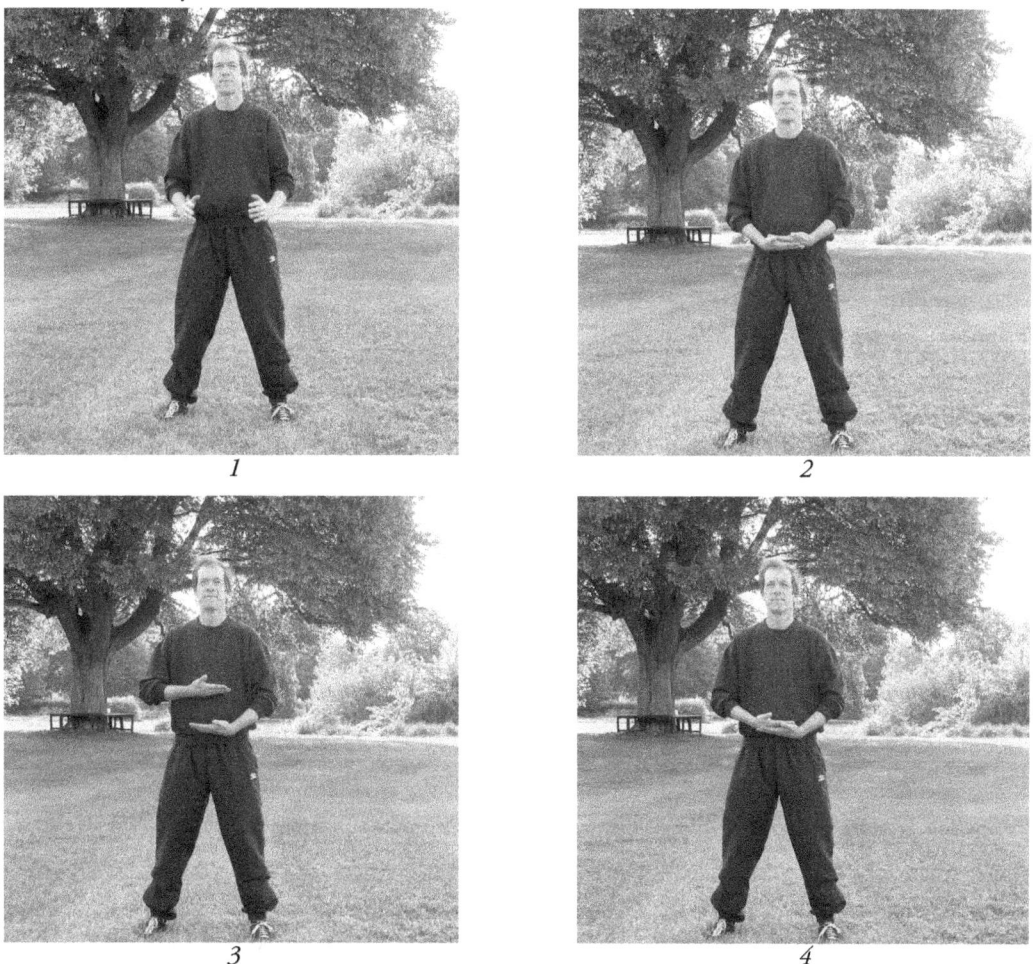

1

2

3

4

Qi Gong

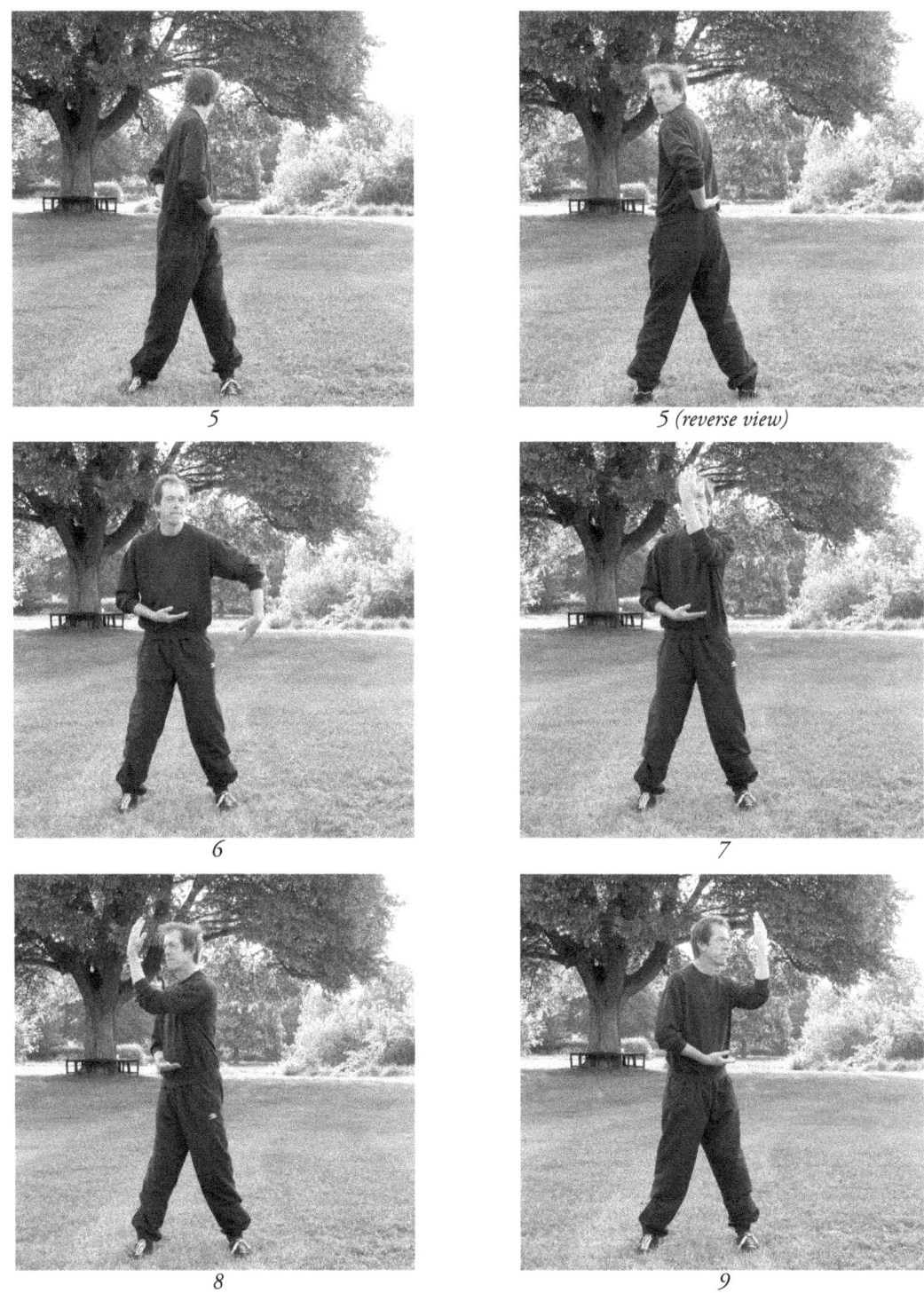

5

5 *(reverse view)*

6

7

8

9

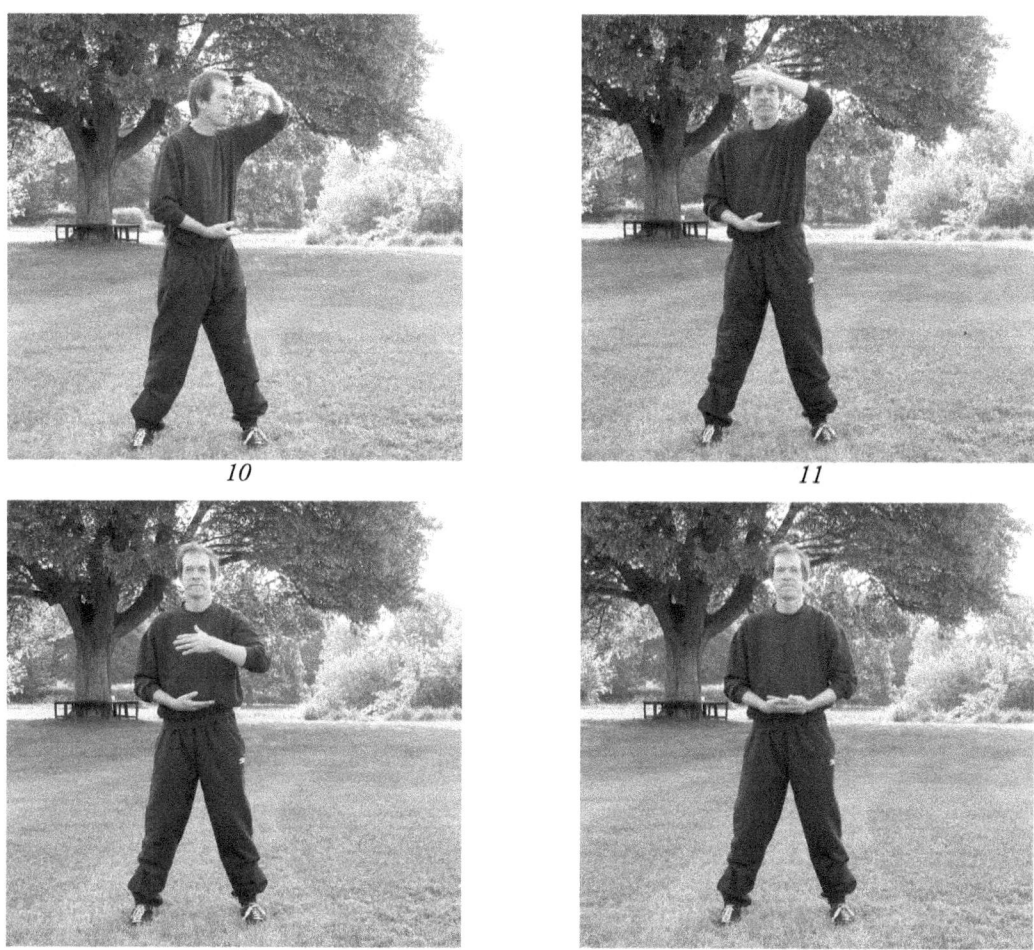

10

11

12

13

No.5

LEG MERIDIANS

The weight is shifted onto the right foot in the starting posture, breathing in as you step out at a 45 degree diagonal with the left foot.

Simultaneously the hands form a triangle shape with the tips of the thumbs and forefingers touching, and are brought up just under the left armpit (axilla). (1, 2, 3)

Maintaining the triangle, bring the hands down the side of the body, exhaling. Pause at the hip. (4)

Breathe normally as you feel the energy at this position. Inhale, then bend forward as you draw the hands down the left leg with the exhale. (5, 6) Left hand goes down the left side, right palm down the right side, fingertips still connected.

Continue over the sides of the feet. When you get to the toes the fingers can separate although the thumb tips are connected. (7)

Inhaling, bring the hands back up the sides of the leg. The right hand then separates and goes past the groin to press on the Dan Tien, while the left hand goes around the back to press the Ming Men. (8, 9) (Photo 10 demonstrates reverse view).

Exhale, swinging both arms out and forward, palm up, and stepping the left foot back. Inhale energy through the hands. (11)

Now step out 90 degrees with the left foot, toes pointing to the left, and again the hands form a triangle, but this time at the hip. Pause to feel the energy there. (12)

Exhale as both hands come down the outside of the leg as you bend forward over it, around the outside edge of the foot, the toes and inside edge of foot as you start breathing in, then up the inside of the leg, and past the groin. (13, 14, 15, 16)

Straighten up, foot back in position facing forward, hands in triangle form with fingers pointing down and pressing on the Dan Tien. (17)

As usual, relax and repeat on the other side.

On the first part of the exercise as you've stepped out at a diagonal, the hands are said to have a 'dredging' effect as the right hand goes down the inside of the leg, then the left hand goes up the outside of the leg, both movements being against the natural flow of energy.

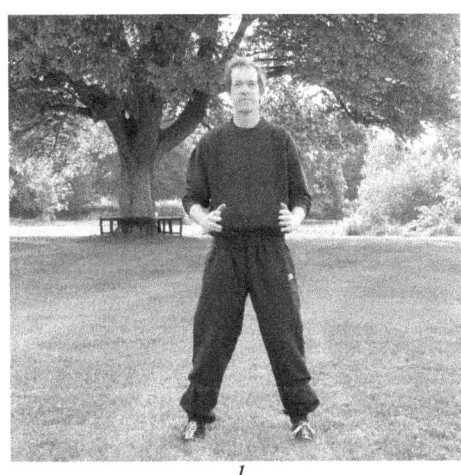

1

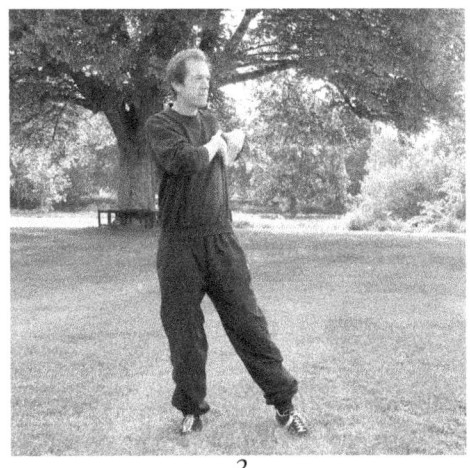

2

The Yuan Qi Exercises

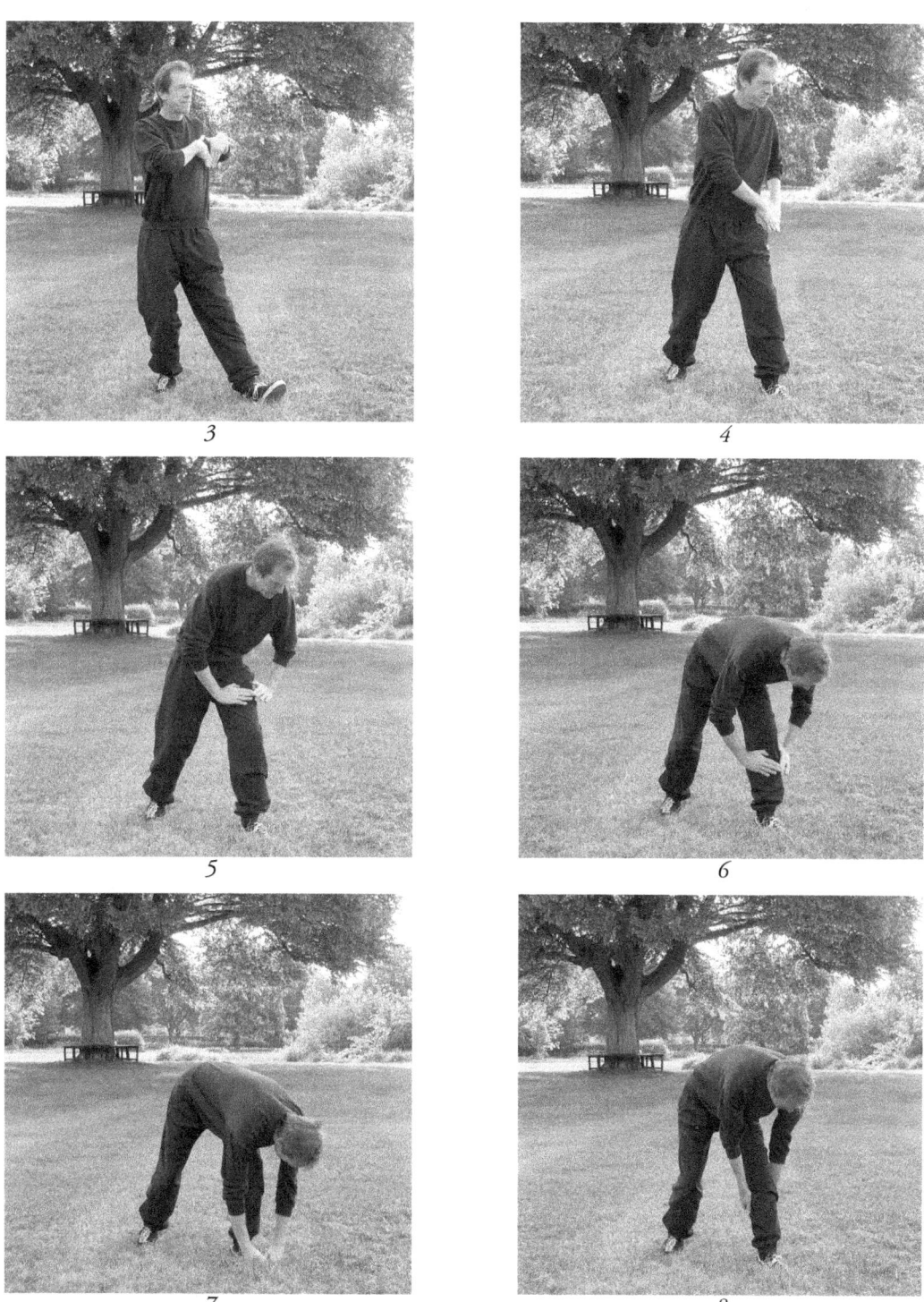

Qi Gong

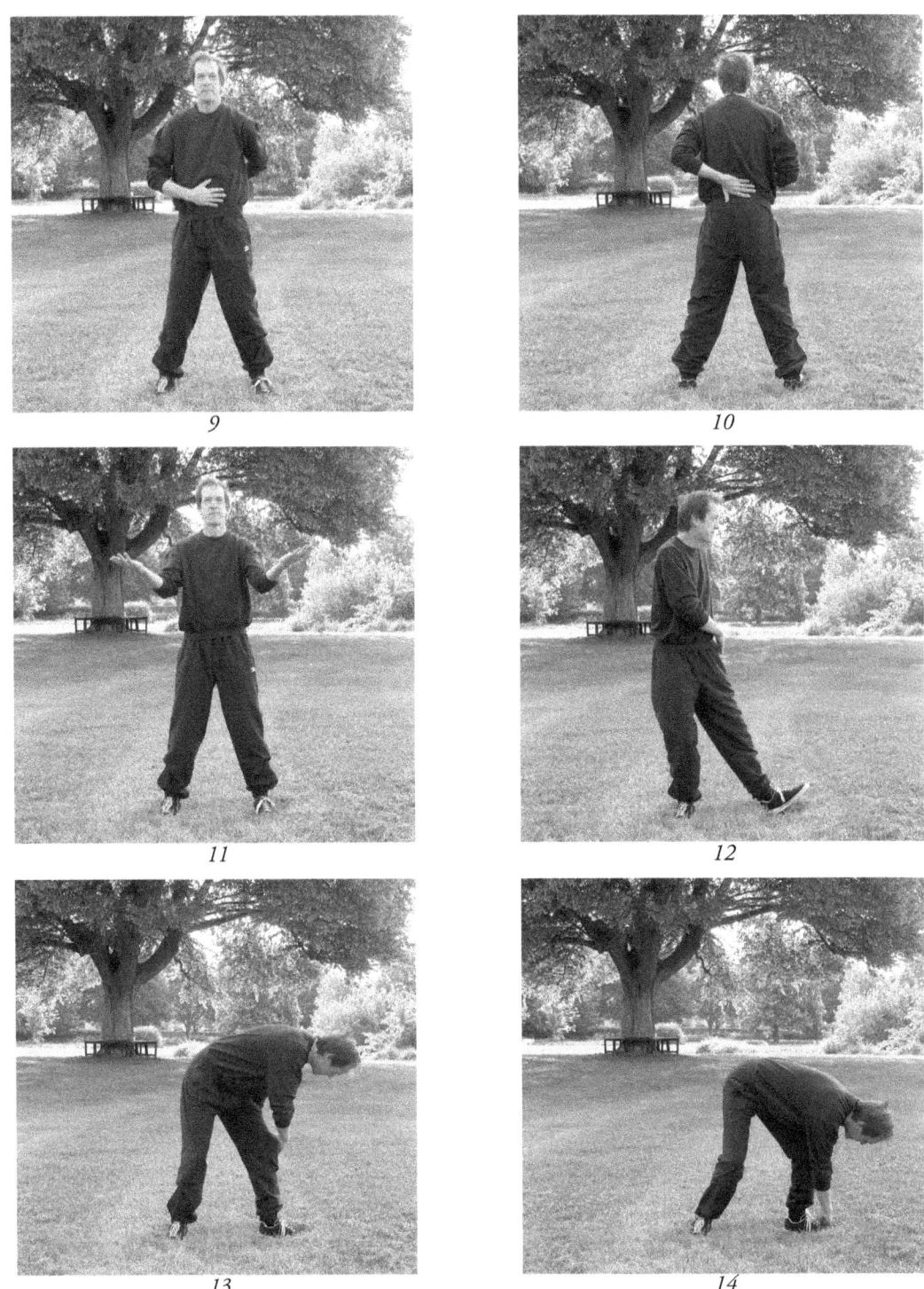

The Yuan Qi Exercises

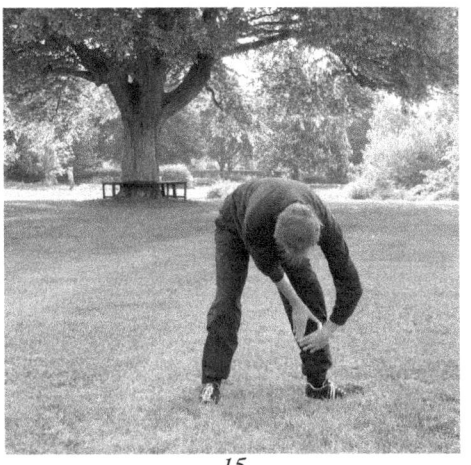
15

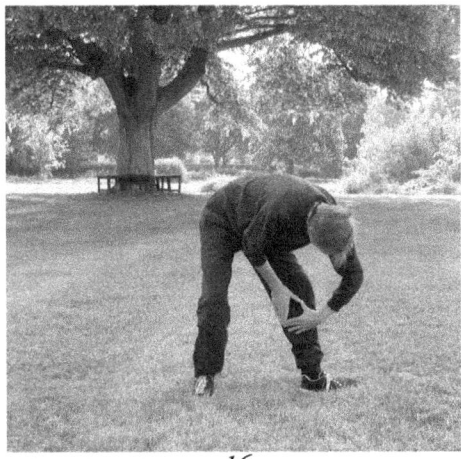
16

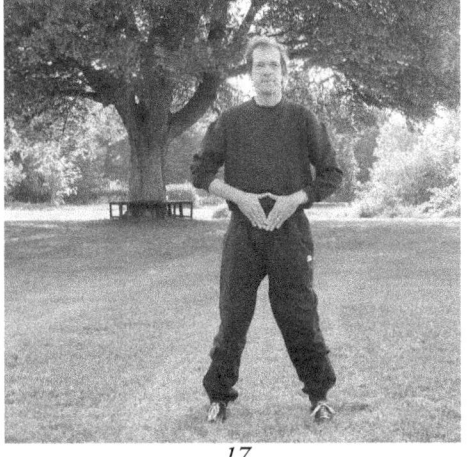
17

No.6

THE BELT CHANNEL

For this exercise you simply maintain the opening stance.

Three circles are formed (in fact as a separate Qi Gong this posture is sometimes known as the Three Circle Stance).

One circle is made by the space between the thumbs and index fingers of both hands. One by the curve of the arms, as if holding a large beach ball. And the third is around the waist.

This third circle is the Belt or Girdle Channel, the Dai Mo, and you can think of it

Qi Gong

as lying a little beneath the skin.

Imagine that energy runs around this circle, beginning from the left kidney area and proceeding past the right, around the front of the body and back to its starting point. This is one round.

Make 9 rotations, then reverse the cycle from the left side, around the front, past the right kidney and back to the left.

Just breathe deeply with this exercise; you might find the breath co-ordinating with the circularity of the energy flow.

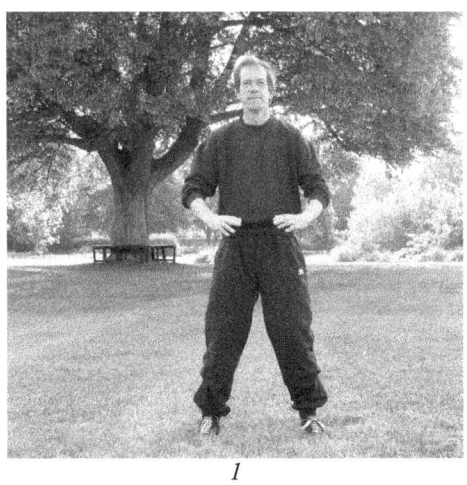
1

No.7

THE LARGE CIRCULATION OF QI

From the Holding the Ball posture, turn the feet to point at 45 degree angles outward. Then, as in the start of the Arm Meridians exercise, place the back of the left hand on the palm of the right held in front of the Dan Tien. (1, 2)

Inhaling, draw the right hand out and above the left, exhale as you press it down onto the left palm. (3, 4) Breathe naturally for the rest of the exercise and try to keep the moving palm facing up all the time.

Turning the waist to the left, bring the left hand around the side, fingers pointing in, then press the LI4 Point onto the Ming Men, as you look behind. (5)

Now bring the hand out and around, fingers pointing outward, describing the arc of a horizontal circle, but also spiralling slightly up as the back of the hand comes over the

The Yuan Qi Exercises

Third Eye Point and you tilt back the head and waist. Your weight follows the direction of the hand. (6, 7, 8, 9)

The hand continues to arc around back over to the left, weight following to the left foot, then it arcs around the front and over to the right shoulder, connecting the edge of the hand to the shoulder. (10, 11)

Keeping it there, bring your weight over the left foot, then back to the right. (12, 13)

Release the hand from the shoulder, and it arcs around the front again. (14)

Then bring your weight over the left foot as you tilt back to look up at the back of the hand, once more over the Ying Tang Point. (15)

It arcs down and around in front of you again, weight shifting accordingly to right foot then left as you bring the LI4 point back into contact at the Ming Men Point, looking once more behind. (16, 17, 18)

Bring the hand past the waist, fingers pointing inward and palm still up, breathing in, over the right palm. (19, 20)

Breathe out as you press it down onto the right hand. (21)

Adjust your feet to point forward and relax. (22)

Repeat on the other side.

This is the most difficult exercise of the set to explain, and probably to perform, but if you follow the instructions step by step and persist it will become easier. This one definitely displays its Bagua origins. My teacher called it the 'Plate' exercise; imagine you are holding a plate, like a waiter, as your hand turns around the body, keeping the palm pointing up.

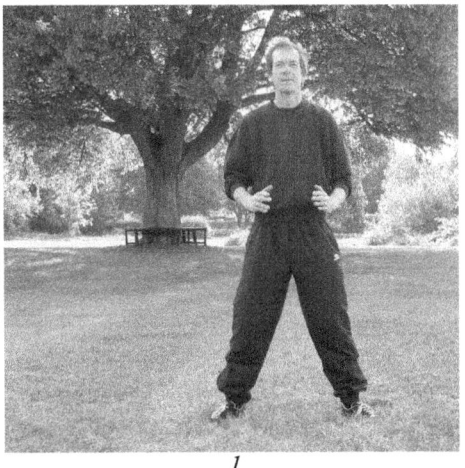

1

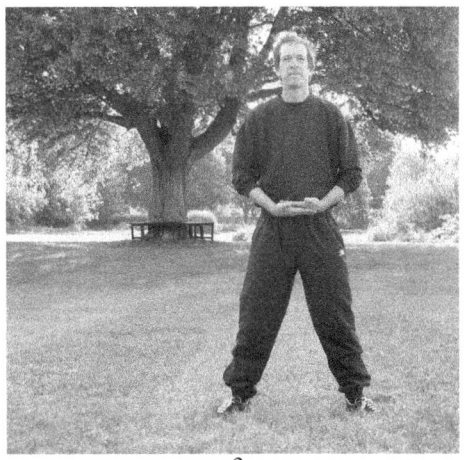

2

Qi Gong

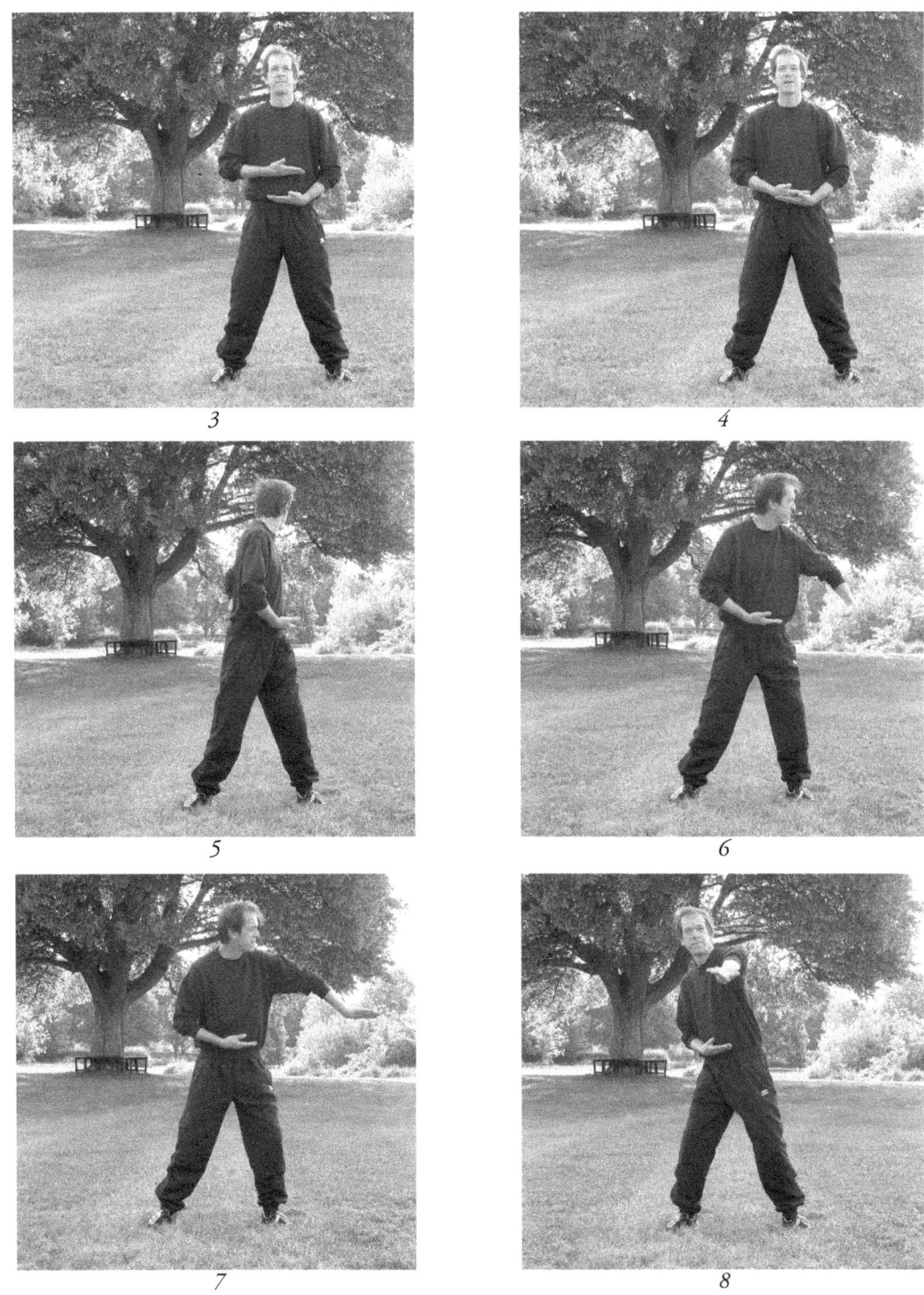

The Yuan Qi Exercises

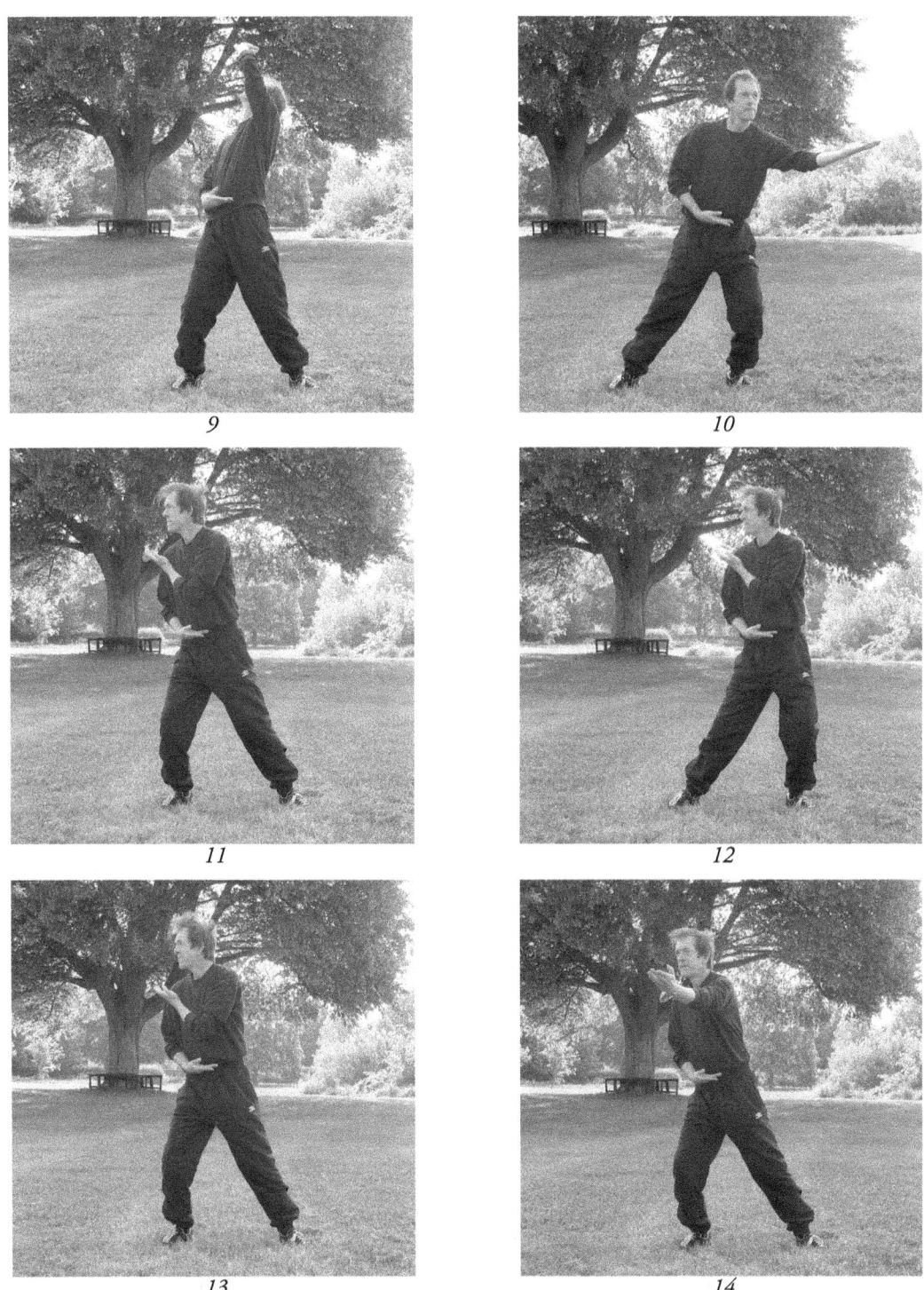

Qi Gong

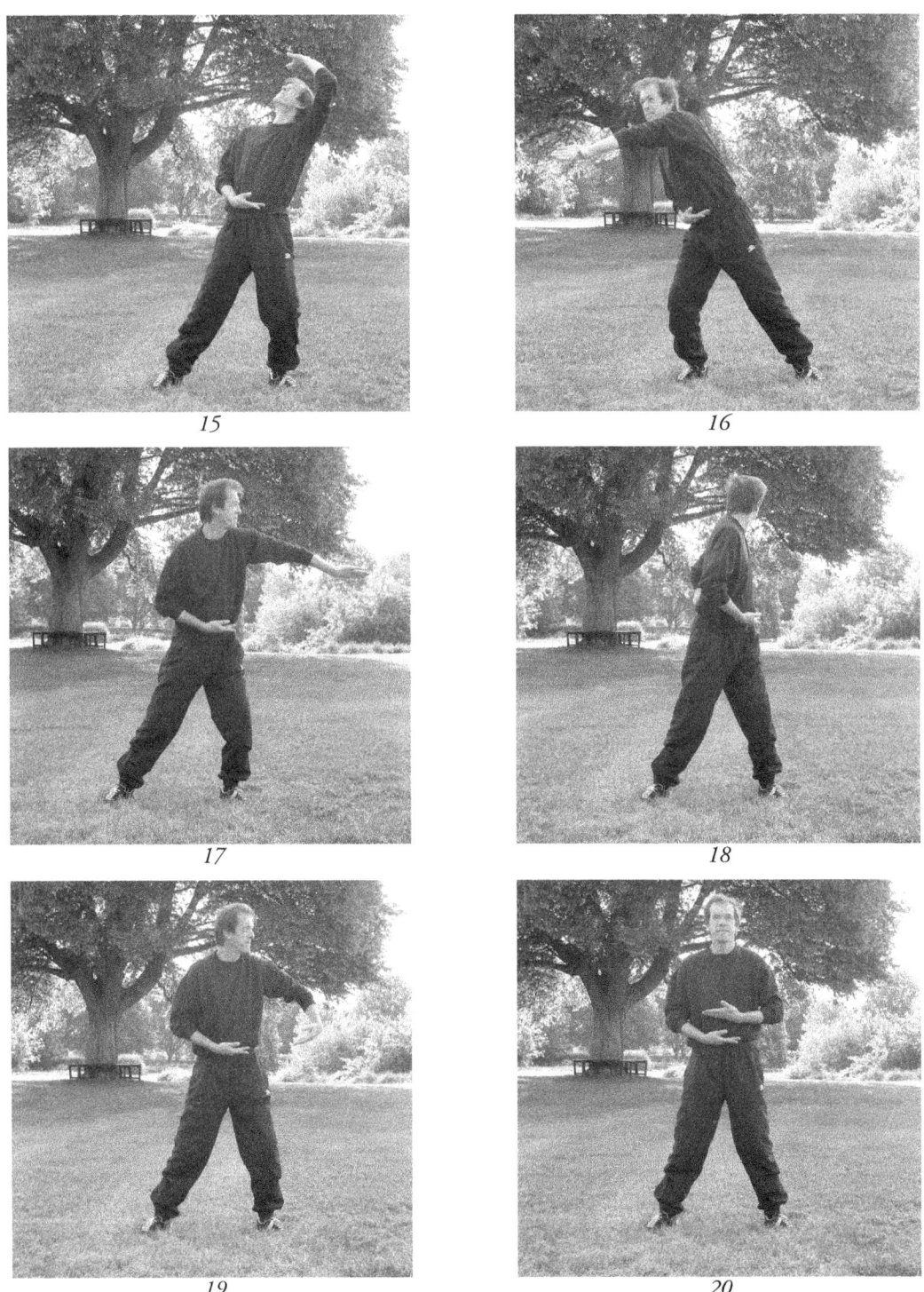

The Yuan Qi Exercises

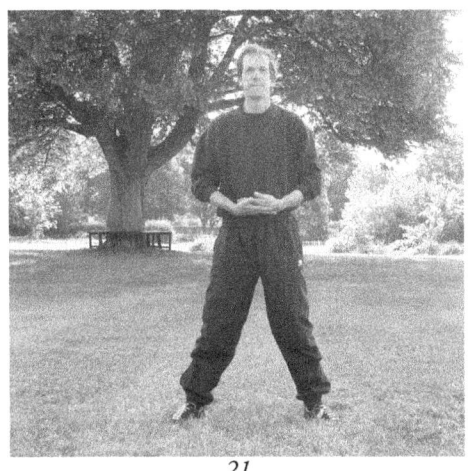
21

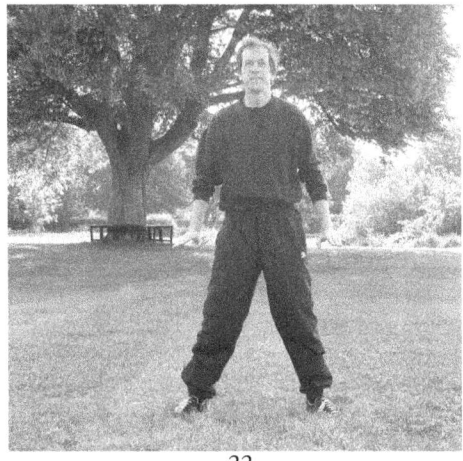
22

No.8

ZHANG FU

From the usual start, bring the arms out to the sides, breathing in, palms up at about shoulder level and imagining you are collecting Heavenly Qi into the Heart Centre and down to the Dan Tien. Breathe out. (1, 2)

Turn the hands to face down and lower the arms slightly, imagining now on breathing in that you are collecting Earth energy through the palms to the Dan Tien. Breathe out again. (3)

Now with the inhalation bring the hands inward, fingers connecting at the level of the Third Eye Point.

Breathe out and down to the Dan Tien. Keep the hands in place. (4)

Breathe normally as you imagine the Ba Hui or Crown Point at the top of the head opening. Take your time. When you are ready, inhale energy as a white light down through the body as the hands lower to the level of the Dan Tien. (5, 6)

Keep the movement going as you exhale, bringing the hands down the legs, angled slightly on the outside, and press on the tops of the feet. (7, 8)

With the inhalation, bring the hands back up the legs, slightly on the inside this time, to form a triangle shape at the Dan Tien. (9, 10)

Press then relax on the exhale. (11)

Qi Gong

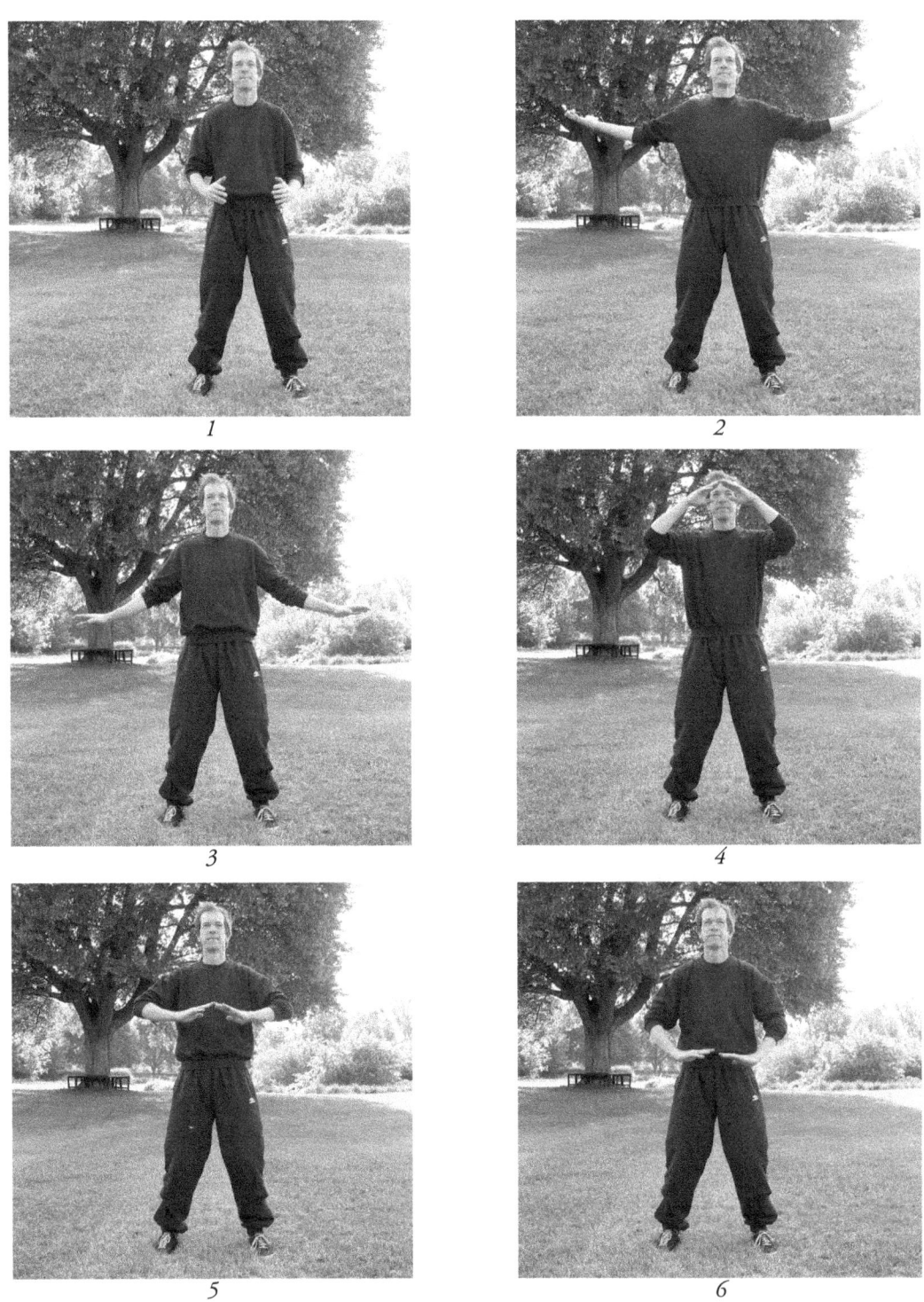

The Yuan Qi Exercises

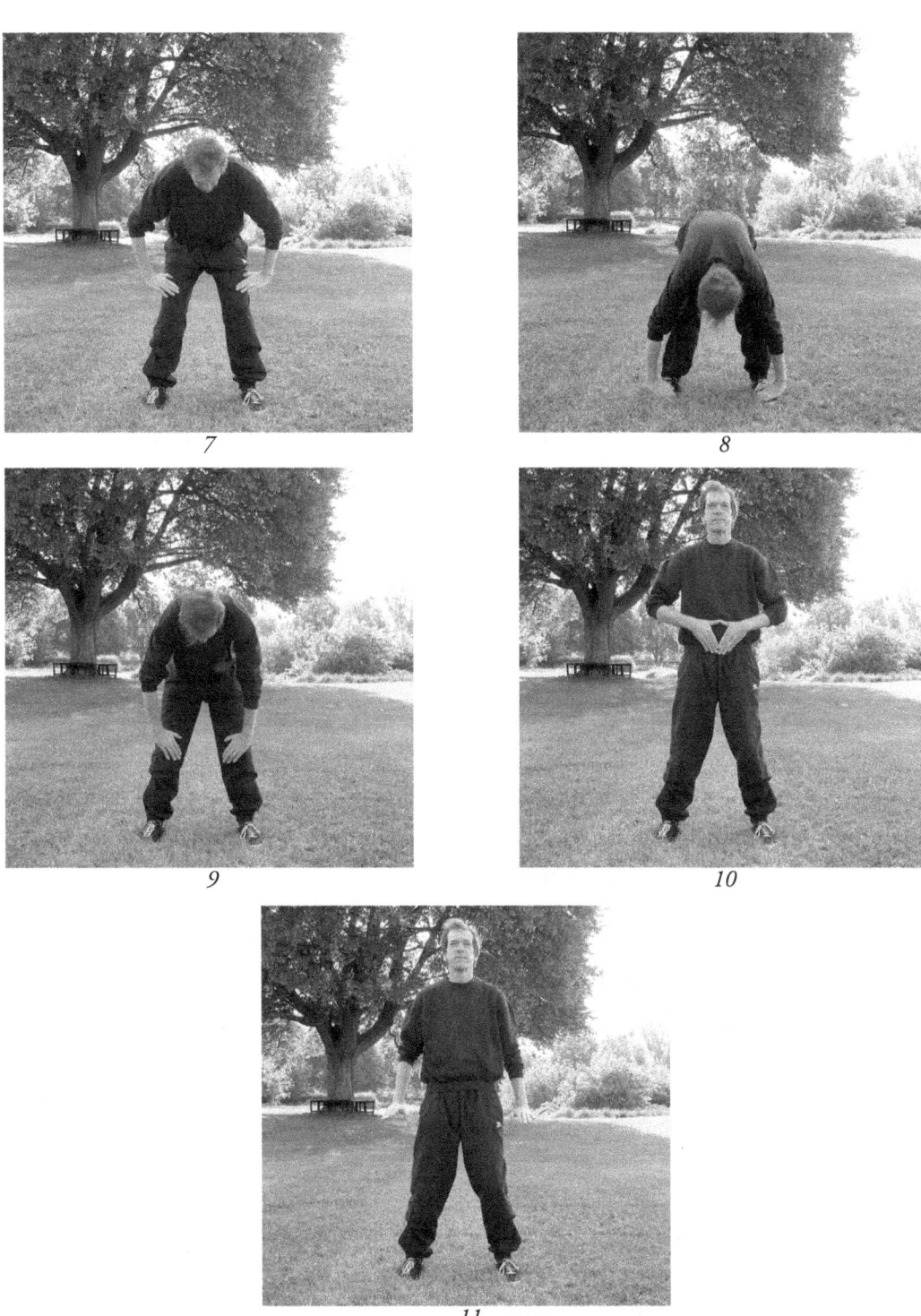

CONCLUSION

1. Spiralling Qi from the Dan Tien.

Still standing in the basic stance, place the right hand on the Dan Tien, left in a loose fist hanging at your side. (1)

Imagine energy spiralling out from the Centre, 36 increasingly large spirals but not higher than the diaphragm. Then reverse the spirals so they become progressively smaller, again 36 times.

Men should first spiral the energy out in a clockwise direction (if you think of a clock face being flat on your abdomen as you look down on it), then reverse spiralling in, anti-clockwise.

For women the order is reversed, anti-clockwise spiralling out and clockwise back in. This is due to the Yin/Yang energy differentiation between male and female.

2. Energy Circuit.

Next, sit on the floor with shoes off, hands together in a prayer position, elbows resting on the knees, and the soles of the feet together. This creates an energetic circuit. (2)

Imagine energy circulating around the Small Orbit, and then around the Large Orbit (down and up the legs and arms).

To finish concentrate on the Dan Tien.

3. Bone Marrow Washing. (Xi Sui Jing).

Still sitting, place your feet flat on the floor, elbows remain resting on the knees and hands in the prayer position.

Visualize energy being drawn up into the bones of the feet and spiralling through them.

Progress to the hips, pelvic area, coccyx, sacrum, spinal column, over the skull, down the sides of the head to the jaw, down to the clavicle, sternum and ribs, back through the ribs to the sternum and clavicle again then down the arms, hands and fingers.

To conclude, concentrate on the Ming Men.

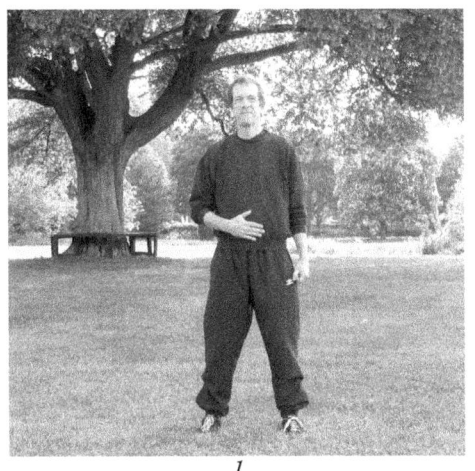
1

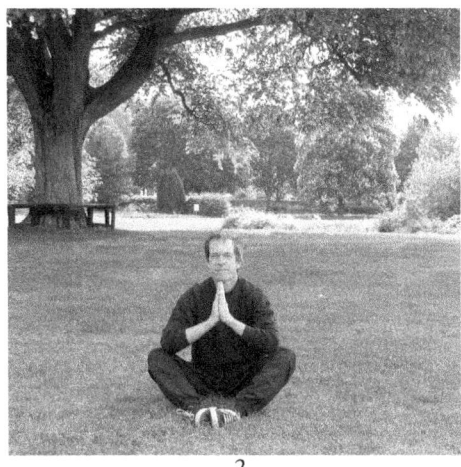
2

4. Qi Self Massage (An-Mo).

Rub your hands together until the palms are warm. Then gently massage the fingers from knuckles down to fingertips.

Massage around the temples, above the ears to the back of the head, up to the crown, down to the eye-brows and back to the temples 3 times.

Tap gently all over the scalp with your fingertips.

Massage over and under the eyes with the edge of the forefinger.

With the thumbs, massage up either side of the nose to the hairline and down.

With one hand going up as the other goes down, alternate rubbing the palms simultaneously over the face.

Massage around the ears, and also flick the edges of the ears.

Rub the kidneys in outward then inward circles.

Points massage - outside of the knee just below the top of the fibula is Gall Bladder 34, which generally relaxes the muscles. Stomach 36 is located about three finger widths below the knee on the front of the leg, on the outer side of the tibia, and is credited with a variety of effects including strengthening the immune system. GB40 at the front lower edge of the outer ankle is another muscle relaxing point, and Liver 3 between the first and second metatarsals helps to calm emotions.

Massage generally with stroking movements outside and inside the lower leg.

Massage the toes; the two points either side of the nails, on the big toe, the second, fourth and little toes, leaving out the middle one (no meridians terminate at the middle toe).

Rub the soles of the feet with the palms, and to finish hold the K1 point with the thumb on each foot.

12. WALKING

'I wish to speak a word for nature'. Thoreau.

I have a couple of relatives in excellent health whose sole (no pun intended) exercise regime consists simply of taking long walks. Walking is such a good exercise due to the Yin/Yang rhythm having a balancing effect right through the body from the feet up, following the idea of the well-known 'cross-crawl' exercise; because our neurology is contralateral or cross-patterned, movement that consists of one leg going forward at the same time as the opposite side's arm helps to balance the brain's two hemispheres, a cerebral connection that affects coordination and other physical qualities such as perception. This kind of practice has also been credited with helping to restore nerve function in some cases of trauma. There are variations of on-the-spot cross-crawl such as touching an elbow to the other side's knee, and even seated versions.

Various overall health benefits have been associated with regular daily periods of walking, and studies have found it can even reduce the risk of dementia, Alzheimer's, diabetes and heart disease, and can increase bone health and prolong life expectancy. As a cardio-vascular exercise walking at a brisk pace conditions the lungs and heart, and helps strengthen and improve muscular endurance without the potential for injury that jogging has. It also provides a tissue-cleansing effect.

A further effect in walking as exercise is that the reflex points on the soles are massaged, especially by the variable surfaces if you take a ramble in the countryside. Maintaining good posture, the aspects of physical alignment that apply to the standing position, is important. A conscious, rhythmic pace is important rather than just wandering.

Regarding the biomechanics of walking, the centre of mass of the body is raised to its highest point as the leg assumes a vertical position, with the supporting knee straightened. There is an exchange of the kinetic energy of forward movement with an increase in potential energy. Technically it is comparable to a pendulum motion.

Meditative walking can be simply walking whilst being aware, without trying to change anything about how you walk. In this way it provides an interface between body and mind attentiveness. The formal kinds of meditative linear walking are the type found in Tai Chi, where we contemplate our balance and become more aware of how our weight is adjusted through stepping. A typical Tai Chi exercise in this respect is to lift a foot, feeling how stable you are balanced on one leg, step forward very slowly onto the heel, and roll your weight forward until the foot is flat on the ground. Slowly lift the heel of the rear foot until it is poised on the toes and then lift it off the ground and step up to place the toes by the instep of the other foot. Pause, taking a deep breath in and out, then step out with that same foot you have just stepped up with, and go through the whole routine again, heel down, rolling the weight forward, and repeat.

At each step you are sinking your weight down without placing stress upon the knees. The knees should not project over the toes when you have the foot placed flat on the ground. Breathe out as you step out, in as you step up. It's probably not recommended to perform this kind of meditative walking in the local High Street.

Maintaining a focused state of mind as you walk is of course a more challenging exercise than remaining still, because of the distractions imposed by a shifting environment and the myriad conditions of space and encountered obstacles to negotiate.

It can be seen as a discipline in learning to compartmentalize experience, a fundamentally necessary property. Through compartmentalizing, challenging events and situations can be isolated and not become issues of obsession. To improve this faculty, we can isolate individual components such as the breath, the footsteps, and so forth, giving each our full attention in turn. We could otherwise turn our attention entirely to the surroundings, again by component, i.e. the ground, buildings, sky etc. The focus is ideally maintained for as long as possible. A progression is to concentrate on two elements simultaneously.

If you take a look at the soles of your shoes they might reveal something about your manner of walking, the areas of most wear indicating your weight distribution. I've seen some people actually walking on the sides of their shoes, instead of the soles, without being aware of it. Not good.

The foot is a complex structure having 26 bones and 33 joints, with around 50 muscles. There's an entire science devoted to gait analysis. With the development of photography it became possible to see details of animal movement that were not previously detectable by direct observation, such as the way horses gallop (captured in the famous set of photographs by Eadweard Muybridge). Video recordings of sports professionals in action help them develop their technique by an analysis of the way they move.

Reflexology works on a holographic principle that a part of the body, in this case feet and hands, can act as a model for the whole. Reflex points correspond to organs and systems. When I worked as a practitioner we used to combine it with the Metamorphic technique as the two therapies complement each other. The Metamorphic Technique is unique in working on a temporal aspect, the gestation period, through the spinal reflexes on the inner edges of the feet, the thumb sides of the hands, and the back of the head. It can be related to the idea of Prenatal energy.

The toes are terminal (Yang) and origination (Yin) points for six meridians. The Spleen and Liver meridians start on the big toe, and the Kidney meridian K1, the Yong Quan (Bubbling Spring or Well) on the sole of the foot (this point is good to massage for improved sleep and appetite. It can also restore consciousness).

The Stomach meridian ends on the second toe, the Gall Bladder on the fourth, and the Bladder meridian on the little toe. The tips of the toes signify the time of conception in the Metamorphic paradigm, the spinal reflexes are indicative of the time in the womb, and the inner ankles express the time of birth.

We don't usually pay much attention to our hard-working feet, and they probably deserve better treatment than they are given. They support and balance us on a relatively small surface area, providing our foundation and connecting us to earth. They also communicate something about our identity as we initiate movement with a step. 'Best foot forward', 'One small step for Man' and 'Knowing where you stand' are all expressions of our 'root' communication with the world, contributing to the forging of identity. Making a stand.

'Walking the Path' is invariably used as a metaphor for spiritual practice. Philosophers such as Jean - Jacques Rousseau have extolled the value of meditative walking (see his 'Reveries of the Solitary Walker'), and Henry David Thoreau's essay, succinctly titled 'Walking', became a seminal work in the environmental movement.

Because the foot supports the body it is representative of the foundation of our self, the spirit or soul. The footprint has a significance as an imprint of purely being, an example is the reverence accorded the footprints supposedly left by the Buddha at several locations. This form of essential signature, the quintessence or recognition of existing, is exemplified by the hand and footprints set in concrete by Hollywood personalities.

As a mark of respect, shoes are taken off when entering some sanctuaries and places of worship, separating the mundane from the sacred. The act of washing the feet is given particular importance in the Bible, as a symbol of cleansing the way, clearing the detritus of old paths that have been trod in order to renew the wayfarer, rather than as an act of humility that it is often interpreted as.

By walking on a natural surface we get back in touch with our own ground experience.

Tarmac surfaces disconnect us because they are for one thing smooth, and so we do not receive a variable condition of pressure upon the complex map of reflexes on the feet. The ancient Taoists were certainly more 'in touch' with the world than we are, with our feet not even connected to the earth but suspended from it by artificial surfaces.

There is an often quoted remark by Chuang Tzu that 'The breathing of the true man comes from his heels' (the chen-jen or true human has realized truth within him or herself, attaining the freedom that is the Tao). The experience is comparable to walking on a sunny day in the countryside, taking in the fresh air and feeling a sense of connectivity with the environment as you walk.

13. CIRCLE WALKING

'When you walk the circle for a time, the Hsien become present'. A Tao-shih.

As the circle is a natural organic form to follow, humans have instinctively pursued circular forms in numerous activities. Sitting and dancing around a fire would have been one of the primal means to establish a sense of community, the Circle Dance being a communal tradition common to a variety of cultures, Celtic, Greek, Eastern European, North and South American Indian, Israeli and Islamic. It was sometimes known as a Sacred Circle Dance when performed for religious or meditative reasons. Mazes and spiral patterns were followed for ritual purposes by pre-Christian peoples. The Crane Dance was a means of solving the riddle of the Greek Labyrinth; the entrance to the underworld and emergence in ceremonial rebirth.

A circumambulation of parish boundaries by members of the community to mark the territory was known as Beating the Bounds, and is still extant in Cornwall. It could have been derived from the Roman Terminalia festival honouring the god of landmarks, Terminus.

There is also the magical practice of drawing a circle around oneself as a means of establishing a protection from obsession when entering altered states of consciousness. The Mandala (Sanskrit for magic circle) is a design used as a focal point in meditation, its circular structure symbolizing the path to individuation or as it could be phrased, Salvation. Its single central point is the goal of self-realization and wholeness.

The true Taoist masters were the Tao-shih, dignitaries of the Tao. Through following the outline of a diagram in a form of a dance, the Taoist master could take possession of the symbol's forces. Very early shamanic practices included following dance patterns that would take the dancer into the sky, such as emulating the pattern of constellations, like the Big Dipper.

The practice of walking the circle is the common training method in Bagua Zhang, or eight trigram palm. As a Taoist Qi cultivation method its aim is to seek union with the natural world, or 'The circumambulation of the Self' as Jung put it, in contrast to seated static meditation where the focus is inward. As the earth rotates around the sun and also around its own axis, so the practitioner is attuned to the greater cycles operating around us, 'a circle whose centre is everywhere and circumference nowhere,' (Liber XXIV Philosophorum).

Dong Hai Chuan, the creator of the Bagua fighting method, was a member of the Quan Zhen (Complete Truth) Taoist sect, which can be traced back to the 8th-century Tang Dynasty, part of the Dragon Gate or Long Men school. This sect practiced circle walking or Rotating in Worship of Heaven (Zhian Tian Zun). Dong's genius was in adapting this meditative exercise to create an extremely effective fighting art. He was taught by two Taoist masters who apparently had him walk around a tree for seven years, then around two trees in a figure 8 for two years. This is indicative of the kind of unquestioning discipline that was required in the typical student/master relationship, not something that is common-place in the Western style of teaching, where pupils tend to want to be given a reason for every action they are asked to take. Arguments can be made for or against either style of teaching. The value of obedience is in preserving a teaching exactly; that of individuality, in reaching forward to new expression.

The encircling of a tree, post or pole is representative of circling the world's axis, or axis mundi, which symbolically connects heaven and earth. Dancing around a maypole is another example, or the use of the Totem pole. It is advised by some masters that if you walk around a tree as a circle walk exercise you should ask its permission; it's a living thing, after all. You might even get into a conversation.

The Taoists repeated mantras as they walked to focus the mind, creating stillness in motion. The pattern they followed was to walk three times very slowly around a circle, and then track an 'S' shape through the centre to continue in a reversed direction around the circle again. The circle therefore looked like the Tai Chi Yin/Yang diagram.

There are many ways of practicing with a variety of stepping techniques. Some of the steps are named after animals, including the Lion Step, which is the natural heel-to-toe method, and the Chicken Step (you can imagine what that looks like). Others are simply and obviously descriptive, such as the Gliding Step.

The size of the circle varies according to the environment, circles with a larger circumference being usual for meditative purposes, smaller circles for the practice of combat orientated movement. Also in the meditative, healing aspect of circle walking, the body is kept open, with the movements being 'large frame', as contrasted to the 'small frame' combat application with the arms making tighter movements closer to the body.

Circle Walking

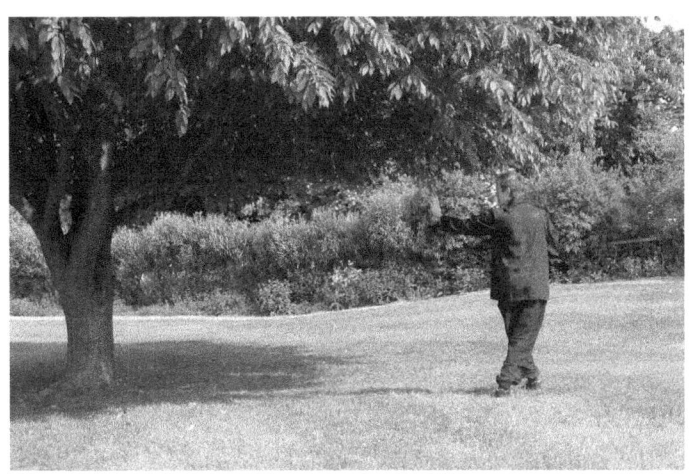

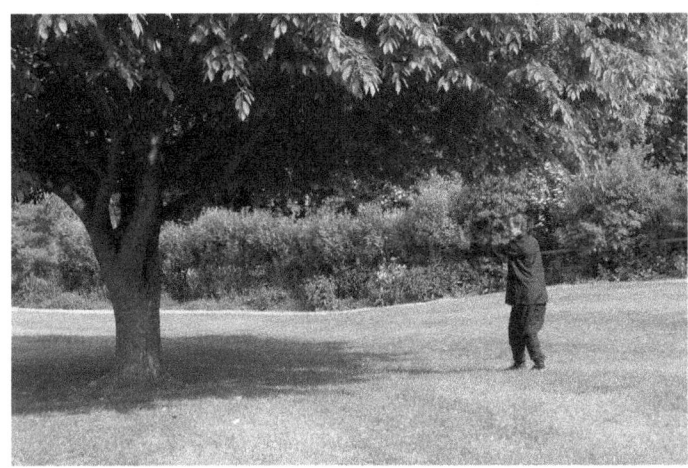

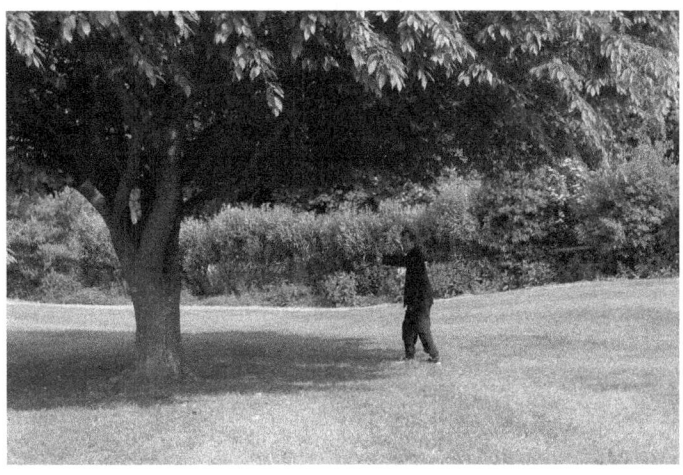

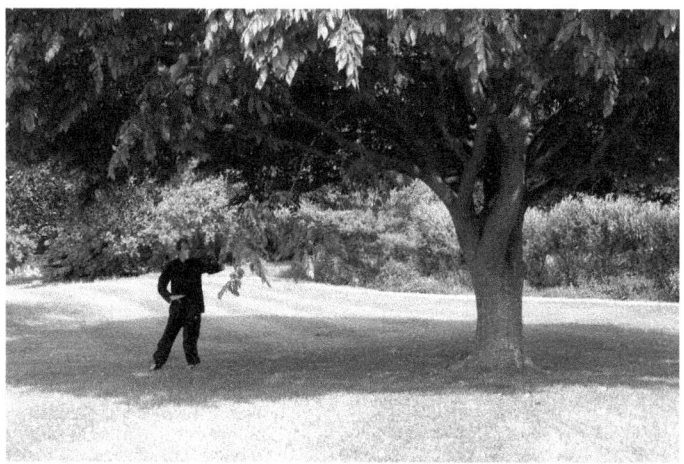

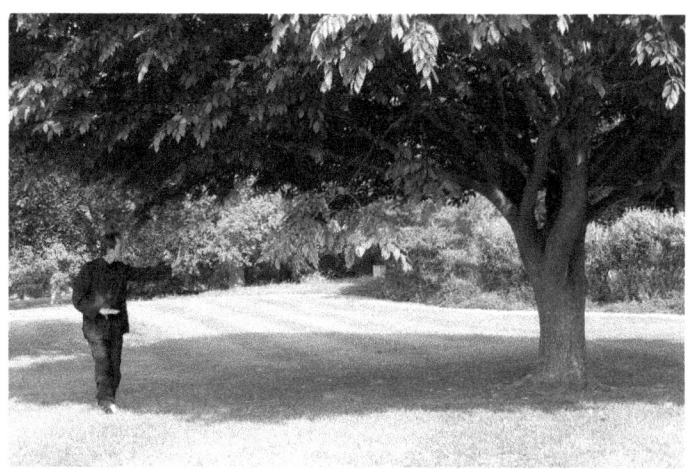

Speed of practice can be slow or fast for the same reasons; fast for a cardio-vascular workout, slow for meditation and balance. A low posture could also be used to strengthen the legs. Some practitioners walk holding weights to build upper body strength and endurance.

Combinations of circles can be used, and walking around one or more trees, or posts. Generally the intention is to feel comfortable and relaxed as you walk, moving smoothly and continuously. There should be a balanced energy flow through the body, stability in the movement, and the mind intent without distraction.

The hips rotate in from the line of the circle 45 degrees to the centre, palm pointing towards the centre, and eyes looking at the centre line, straight ahead and not at the ground. This is why trees or posts are sometimes used, as focus or in fighting training to represent the opponent.

Circle Walking

Look through the gap between the index finger and the thumb, the Dragon's Mouth. Relax the shoulders, particularly the shoulder on the outer side of the circle.

There should be a feeling of conversely exerted pressures, like a torque effect, between the focused palm pressing inward to the circle centre and the other side of the torso pressing or rotating outward. This spiralling action effects the building of energy right through the body and is the source of the great power that can be generated in Baguazhang strikes. A great degree of physical flexibility is also developed by the turning of the waist. The abdominal external and internal oblique muscles and the sacrospinalis are the areas to particularly feel the effect of a prolonged session of circle walking.

I usually advocate walking normally in a relaxed manner at first, at a regular pace, and then slowly building the correct components, naturally from the feet up.

As you walk clockwise around the circle (you could actually draw one on your practice ground for clarity, or else imagine it), the left instep and side of the heel are placed on the external edge of the line of the circumference, followed by the right instep and heel being placed on the inner side of the circle's line as you step forward. For the opposite direction, obviously you reverse the application. The ankles brush as you step.

There are three pairs of co-ordinated relationship that should be borne in mind throughout; the shoulders and hips, elbows and knees, and hands and feet. There are also two 'bows' that activate energy, particularly for the fighting art; across the shoulders and down the spine.

A smooth transition from one direction to the other is made by the feet pointing inward or outward from the circle in a 'pigeon-toed' stance, k'ou pu or Eight Step Stance. It is called this because the feet in that position resemble the Chinese character for the number eight.

A sense of connectivity is made both internally through the structural alignment whilst moving, and externally by a feeling of being integrated with the environment.

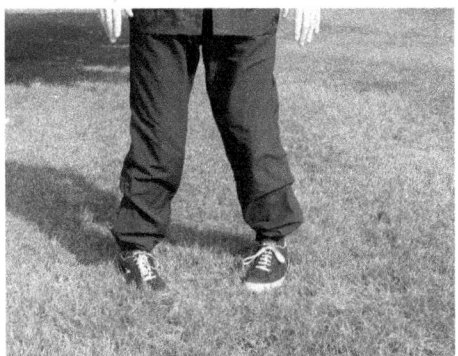

Foot Position

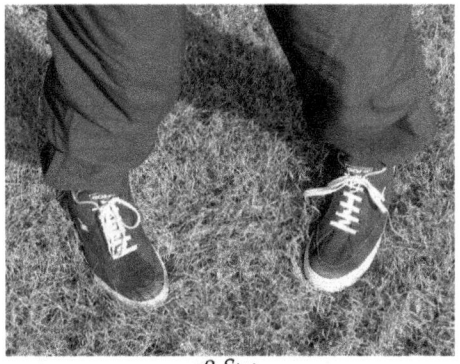

8 Step

Through walking on natural ground (that is, not covered with artificial material) the reflexology points of the feet are stimulated through the gradations in weight transference onto uneven surfaces. You do not focus on any of the energetic point or line aspects such as the meridians, as the energy will move quite naturally where it needs to go without trying conscious manipulation.

You have to establish the biomechanical alignments initially before proceeding too far, or else there will be no progress, or perhaps worse, a false sense of progress.

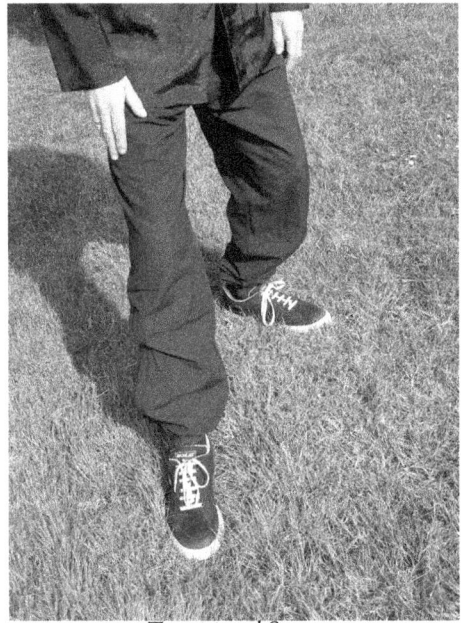
Transitional Stance

14. THE SINGLE PALM CHANGE

'All meditation is conducted in dance'. Mark Hedsel.

After you have practiced the walking exercises for a while, we progress on to the upper body, and the Single Palm Change, or Dan Huan Zhang.

The basic standing posture for Baguazhang in most styles, with minor adjustments, is the Dragon Stance. The head is held up, spine straight, one arm extended with palm in front of the face, looking through the 'Dragon's Mouth' between the forefinger and thumb. The rear guard hand is held opposite the lead forearm, tip of forefinger in line with the Pericardium meridian point 6, about a hand's width below the crease of the elbow. This hand guards the midline of the body. This is the active martial position. For more meditative purposes, the rear hand is positioned opposite the Dan Tien, palm downward, connecting earth energy.

The shoulders are relaxed, elbows dropped. Knees bent, toes of the front foot in line with the toes of the rear foot. Weight sinks down through the feet and is distributed at around 60 per cent on the rear foot, 40 per cent front.

There are various ways to get into the Dragon Posture. Here are two:

1. Stand in a Wu Chi stance with the heels together, feet turned at 45 degree angles. The hands are held relaxed at the thighs and should feel heavy.

Now slowly float them up to the sides and inward, not higher than head level, inhaling, straightening the knees and feeling as though the body is expanding in size. Then bring them down and inwards with the exhalation, the right palm pointing forward, tip of forefinger in line with the nose, left palm at Dan tien level facing down, as you step forward the right foot at the same time as the hands position into place. There are movements of the waist to right then left as you bring the arms up, then back to the right as the hands come down. (1 to 4).

Qi Gong

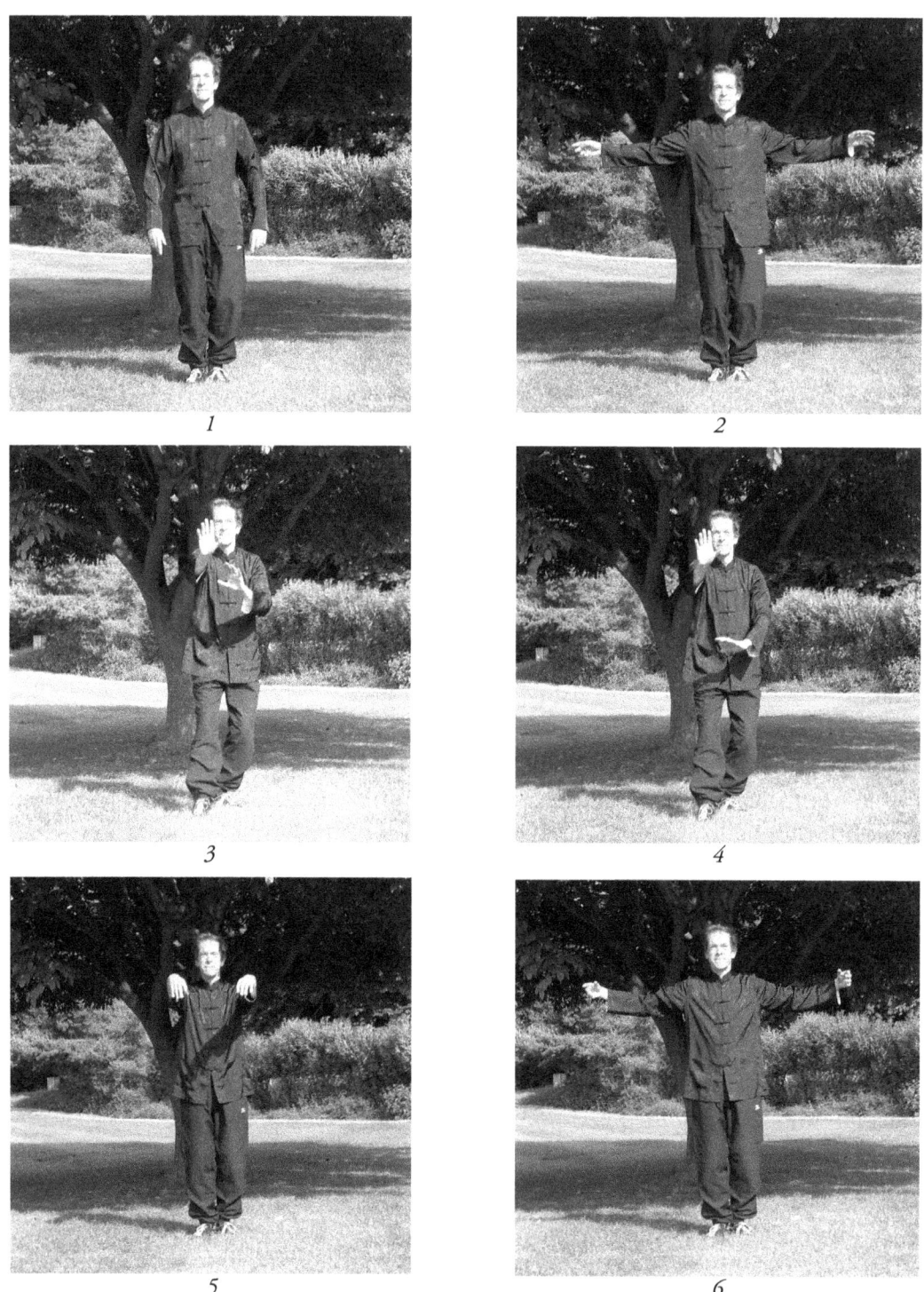

The Single Palm Change

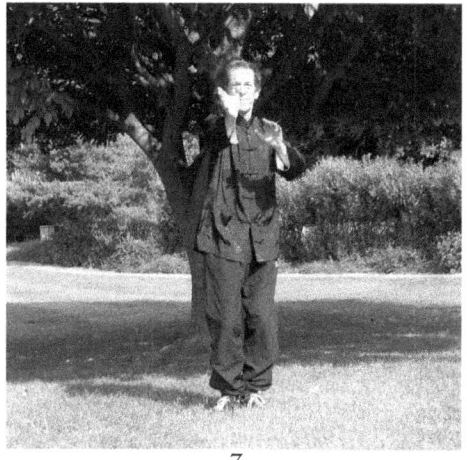
7

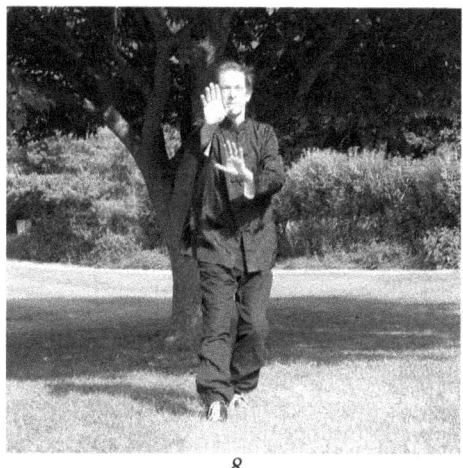
8

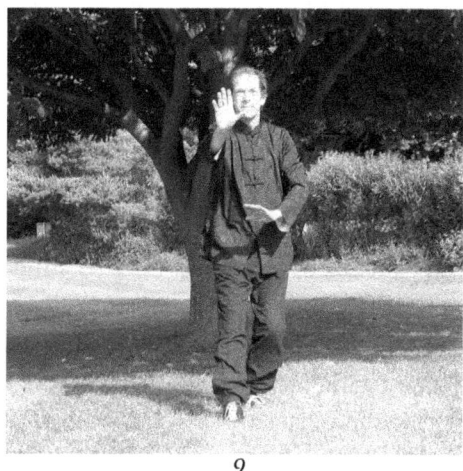
9

2. Another method is to again stand in the Wu Chi posture, as illustrated in figure 1. Begin to inhale and bring the arms slowly up in front, as if pulled up by threads attached to your wrists. Turn the hands so the fingers point toward each other, exhaling. Inhale as you extend the arms out to the sides, and as you exhale bring the arms inward, right palm pushing to the left, left palm pushing toward the right forearm. Simultaneously step forward onto the ball of the right foot. With the pushing inward of the arms the waist has turned slightly to the left, and now it turns back slightly to the right as the right wrist flexes outward with the turn. Both palms then turn to the front as the waist turns again to the left and your front foot is placed flat. (5 to 9).

The waist turning is actually quite subtle in both methods and it should feel like a wave movement. It takes a bit of practice but once everything is co-ordinated and moving together there is an unmistakeable quality of connection. Practice the openings on the other side as well.

The next stage is learning how to change from one arm position to the other side. Stand with the feet and knees together, and bring the arms up into the Dragon Position as explained above but this time without stepping forward. Inhaling, turn the hands palm up, bring the left hand under the right elbow, and slide it forward as the right arm comes back in an arc until the wrists are aligned in the centreline of the body. (10) Exhale as the palms turn outward, the right hand sliding down the forearm of the left as the left arm extends forward. (11)

The shoulders and hips are aligned and at a 45 degree angle at the end of the extension on each turn, so the torso rotates around the body's central axis. That is, with the right arm forward the torso is facing at a 45 degree angle to the left. As the wrists cross, the waist has turned and at this point hips and shoulders are facing directly to the front. With the continuation of the arm movement the body turns to the right 45 degrees. Continue repeating on both sides until it becomes a smooth, flowing action. Next is to continue the movement but out to a 90 degree angle to each side. (12, 13, 14)

The stage after this is a 180 degree turn so the palm points behind you, and then rotating all the way back and around to the rear again, still keeping the feet and knees together and breathing in until the wrists cross, then out each time. Take the 180 degree turn slower and easier, being very careful not to strain your back. Just keep to your comfort zone with this part of the exercise. (15, 16 show front and back views of the posture). Concentrate on the hands to gain a feeling of Qi.

Now we begin to co-ordinate the hand change with stepping, by a step forward with the left foot, integrated with a change from the right palm, forward to the left, stepping back with the feet together as the wrists are crossed, then stepping out with the other foot and hand extended.

You also practice stepping through and back with the palm changes. For example, from a right foot and palm forward stance, step the right foot back past the left as the hands change, so now the left foot is forward and left palm extended. Repeat forward and back.

To practice the movement of the changes as they are performed in the circle, changing direction, step forward with the right foot into a 'pigeon-toed' stance, the right hand coming underneath the left elbow palm up, the left hand palm down by the right shoulder (the foot position as previously explained is known as 8 Step).

Next, step with the right foot forward with the palm rotating out and forward into the Dragon Stance. Now repeat the 8 Step stance on the other side, left foot stepping forward, left hand coming under right elbow palm up, right hand palm down by left shoulder. (17, 18, 19)

The Single Palm Change

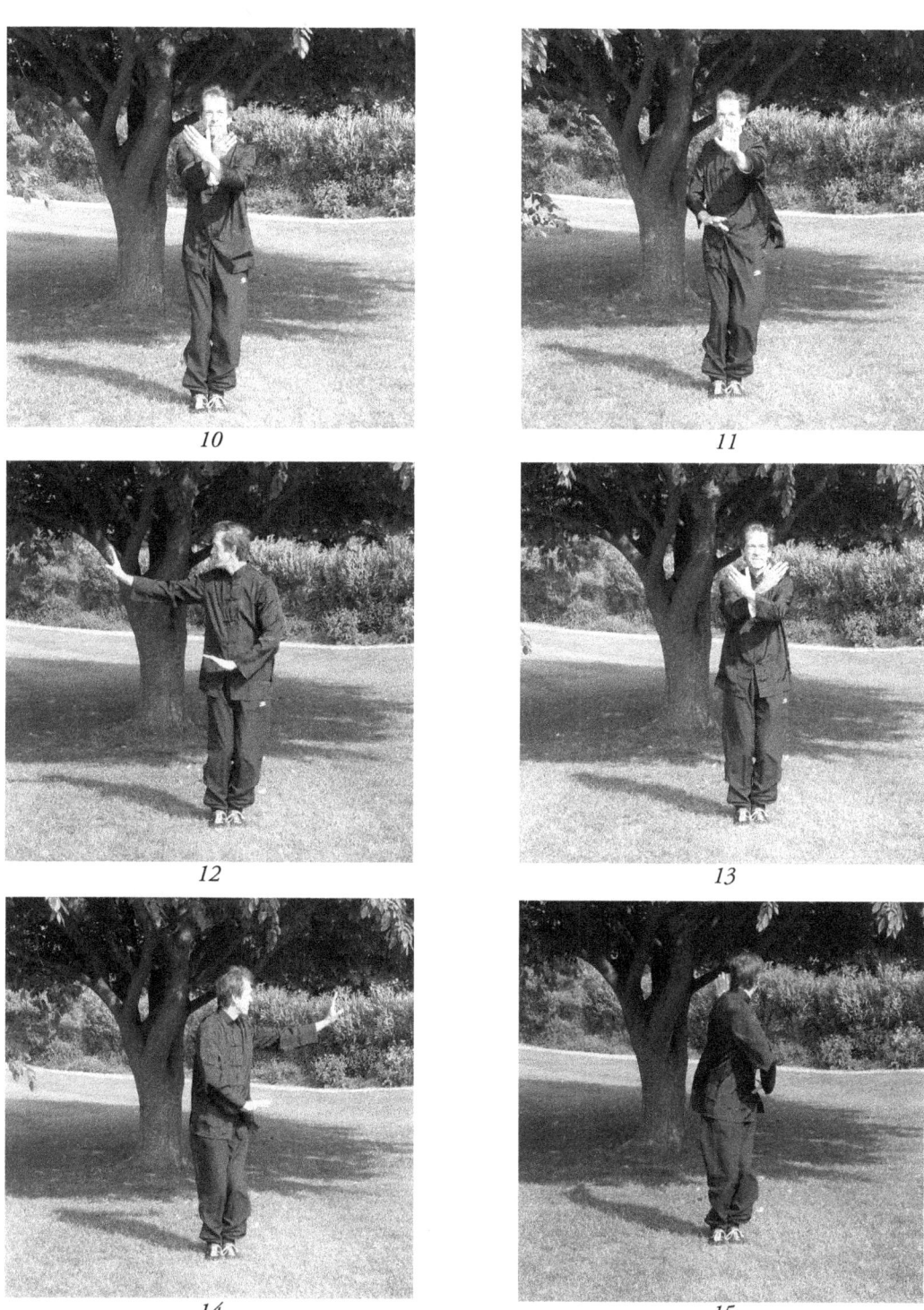

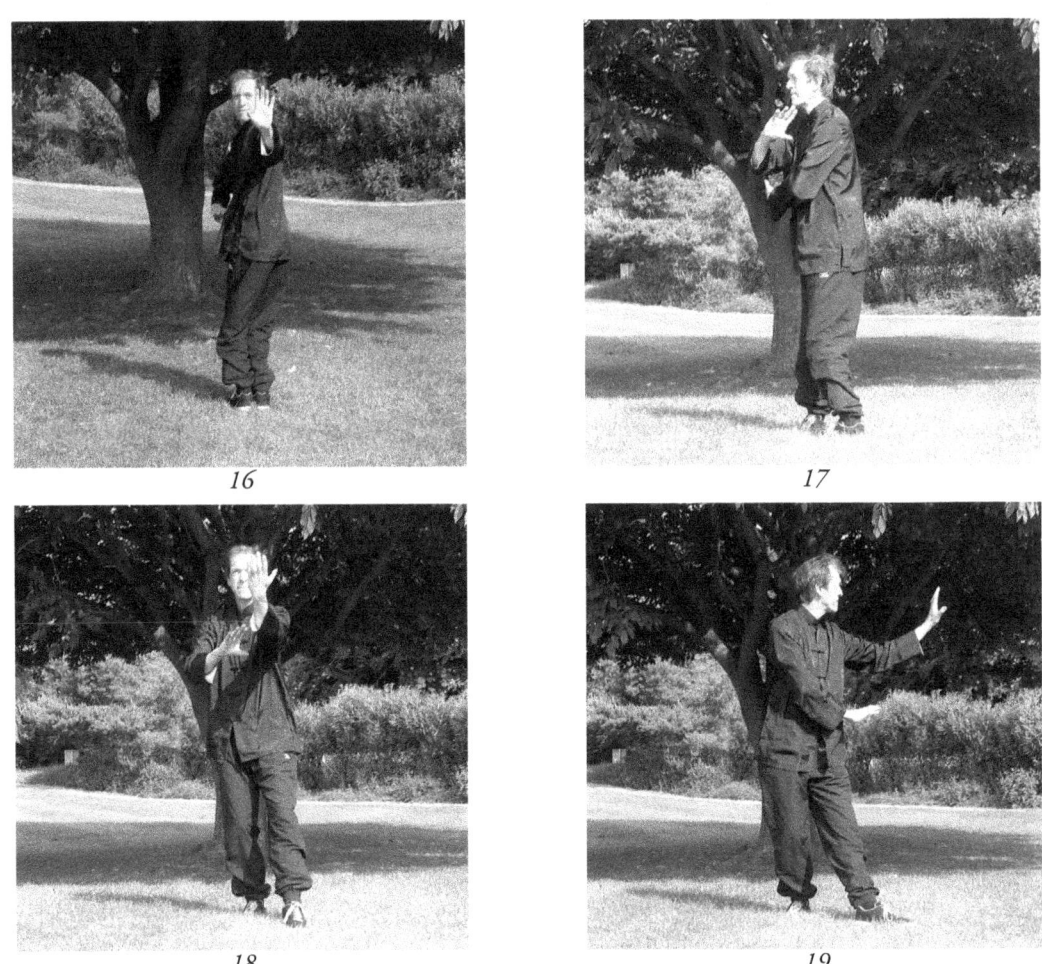

16 17
18 19

THE SINGLE PALM CHANGE AND THE CIRCLE WALK

Beginning from the Wu Chi posture, standing on the circumference of either a marked or imagined circle, heels together and feet pointing at 45 degrees either side of the line, go into the Dragon Stance as explained previously, right hand and foot forward, then step through with the left foot into an 8 Step, facing out of the circle, arms in the Snake Coils Around Tree Position. Release into Palm Change, left hand facing into the centre of the circle as you step around with the left foot and continue walking the circle.

To execute an inside turn, changing from walking anti-clockwise to clockwise, the right foot steps into the 8 Step so you are facing squarely into the centre, forearms crossed. Swing the right palm around to focus into the centre as you simultaneously step to the left with the left foot placed onto the circumference of the circle, and continue walking in a clockwise direction.

An outside turn is basically the same but with the arms describing a larger horizontal arc as you turn. Fundamentally, the upper body position of the Dragon Stance is held as you walk around the circle with the hips rotated at a 45 degree diagonal in toward the centre of the circle and the leading hand focused on the centre. The eyes look straight ahead through the thumb-forefinger space to the centre as you walk. Start with 10 to 15 minutes of walking. Try to keep the head level so you are not bobbing up and down, the body remaining stable as you move.

Between each turn to walking in the other direction, keep the number of circles the same. That is if you walk around three times in one direction turn and walk three times in the other.

The practice of circle walking develops the ability to maintain the physical integrity learnt in the standing practice whilst moving, as well as contributing to general health and flexibility. The spiraling effect utilizes centripetal force to draw energy in, and centrifugal force releasing energy out. It also teaches how to change force and balance smoothly from one side of the body to the other, emphasising co-ordination and connection.

THE HANDS

The Yin meridians that terminate on the fingers are the Lung (ends on thumb), Pericardium (centre of tip of middle finger) and Heart (little finger).

The Yang meridians start on the fingers and are the Large Intestine (index finger), Sanjiao (4th finger), and Small Intestine (little finger). Points on the hands and arms are mostly used for respiratory and circulatory treatment in acupressure therapy.

The Laogong or 'labour palace' is the focal point in the centre of the palm for expressing healing or martial energy.

The Laogong belong to the Pericardium (Heart) channels which regulate Fire energy. The Yongquan points belong to he Kidney channels which regulate Water energy. Together these points are known as the Four Gates.

Generally, the palm facing in or moving in toward the body is a Yin movement; outward direction is Yang. The five digits have also been related to the five elements.

Various gestures and mudras or hand positions are associated with inner states and utilised in a number of ways. They seem to be a profound means to configure emotional response

Crossing oneself is universally recognised even by those with no religious leaning. A more secular example is the V sign, most people having no actual knowledge of its origin or meaning except that it's considered insulting in some countries. Popularly it's thought to be derived originally from the longbowmen at Agincourt, signalling their contempt to the French, who claimed prior to the battle that they would cut off the bowstring-drawing fingers of the English and Welsh archers.

There is also the well-known story of the 'Magical Battle of Britain' during the Second World War, when that fount of occult learning, Aleister Crowley, was allegedly asked to advise Churchill on means to counter the Nazis' use of occult power. Just to recount: Crowley supposedly instructed Churchill to use the V sign as it is a powerful 'warding off' symbol of Apophis or Typhon. It's been noted that as the war progressed to a point where the tide finally turned and the allies began winning, Churchill modified the sign to the more moderate Victory symbol, with the back of the hand turned inward.

The handshake is meant to originate from showing you do not hold a weapon, although this has been contested by some anthropologists. The familiar prayer position as a single hand form signifies the trigram Ken or Mountain in Bagua. The immortal deities of Taoism are associated with mountains, as the word Hsien is written with the characters 'Mountain' and 'Human'. With the hands held together in front of the chest the Middle Pillar/Thrusting Channel is activated. The palm out emergency stop sign is the Bagua 'Fire' palm appropriately.

Some of the unconscious gestures we make are 'tells', to use a poker term, body language revealing our true state of mind. The fingers interlaced and placed over the solar plexus is a protective form, and can be used consciously, as Dion Fortune describes in 'Psychic Self-Defense', to guard against aggressive confrontation, especially with the feet together and placed flat on the floor. This acts to seal the body's energy circuit. Otherwise it can indicate someone who is closed-minded and resisting being influenced.

About the only thing I remember learning from my school physics class was an explanation of the vectors in three dimensional Euclidean space which the teacher demonstrated by a hand gesture, thumb extended laterally in one direction, middle finger at 90 degrees to it horizontally, and the forefinger pointing up. This is also a

The Single Palm Change

hand position taken up subconsciously to, in some order, concentrate the mind; the tip of the forefinger rests on the temple, the middle finger across the mouth and the thumb naturally rests on a point at the side of the jaw known appropriately enough as the 'mind point'.

The meaning of the word temple, from the Latin 'tempus', possibly relates to it being a choice target for a fatal sword blow, due to the visible pulse. It is the position of Gall Bladder 3 as an equally lethal Dim Mak strike. There is also the implication of the right timing for the attack ('temporal'), or alternatively simply relating head space to a temple, as in an abode of spirit or place of worship. The finger on the mouth is indicative of silence, keeping one's own counsel, and a sign of the deity Harpocrates, 'The Babe in the Abyss'. So the mudra implies activity in a void state (Death/Silence), or even the trinity of Time, Space and Event.

Another common mudra that people apply when provoking thought is the steepling of the fingertips together, which coincidentally is an esoteric representation of the cortical surface of the brain.

The Sword Mudra is used in the Taiji jian (straight sword) form, and is used to direct energy, although some experts believe it represents having a dagger in that hand. The first and second fingers are extended with the other two curled into the palm and the thumb folded on top of them. At certain moments in the Form the fingers are actually placed on Lung meridian points, which correlates to the symbolic attribution of the sword to the element of air. This mudra is also used to exorcise evil spirits, and in giving a benediction.

The Tibetan lama mudras are used for meditation and for active effects upon others. In Japan there are a set known as the Kuji Kiri or Nine Cuts, derived from the Tibetan form, which focus three levels of power for each of the three levels of the body.

Baguazhang and the healing and meditative Taoist arts have a variety of hand forms. There are three basic forms for the single palm change;

Lotus palm is made by closing the fingers together, in a layered effect, with the thumb held tightly to the side. The Fan form involves spreading the fingers out wide. I use an intermediary between the two, Tile Hand, with the fingers layered like tiles on a roof, or as in Lotus Palm, but relaxed and open, with the thumb out to the side to open the Dragon's Mouth point, and the palm concave. It's a natural palm to use and facilitates energy flow without taking focus away from the integrity of the rest of the body. There is a Yin/Yang exchange of energy between the hands as you execute the turns around the circle.

The combative reason for employment of the palms rather than fists is the percussive effect a palm strike has upon the internal organs of an opponent.

15. BUDDHIST WALKING

I was intrigued to find that Buddhism has its own tradition of using walking as a spiritual practice, and so I asked Lokabandhu Lokabee, an ordained Buddhist and teacher at the Glastonbury Buddhist Community, if he could give me further information. He has kindly provided the following essay:

In many different ways, walking has always played an important part in Buddhist practice. Here's a very short introduction to four of them.

MINDFUL SLOW WALKING

The first classic practice is simply mindful slow walking. Kamalashila in his classic book 'Meditation: The Buddhist Way to Tranquillity and Insight' says that walking up and down on a straight path, or round and round, can be used as a relaxation exercise, in preparation for meditation, or to become more physically aware by bringing attention to muscular adjustments from the feet up. It both stimulates and has a calming effect. The attention progresses from sensations to the experience of movement through space.

BUDDHIST 'YATRAS'

Mindful slow walking focuses primarily on the body and the ground immediately beneath you - a very detailed and precise approach to awareness. A different approach to walking meditation is to extend the breadth of your awareness to encompass the whole environment and space around you, beneath you and above you, of course including yourself as a part of it. The awareness becomes less precise but much broader and more 'flowing'. The walking is done at a normal pace. Instead of a retreat spent sitting in meditation inside a building, you walk through the landscape in mindful and appreciative awareness of your whole experience, inner and outer. This is what happens on a Buddhist Yatra, Yatra simply meaning 'walk'.

A Yatra may be done alone or in a group. In a group Yatra it is traditional to follow a particular etiquette that helps everyone maintain mindfulness. Participants walk in silence, in single file, beginning and ending each hour-long stretch facing one another in a circle and bowing. At that time there is an opportunity to offer the others any reflections, poems, thoughts etc. a person might wish to share. A leader sets the pace and checks the map; a 'backstop' ensures no one gets lost - everyone else is therefore free to simply walk 'in the moment'. In this way a group might walk ten or more miles through the landscape; a Yatra might last a week or more, with people camping each night.

The European Dharma Yatra has been running since 2001, on which over 200 people from more than 20 countries worldwide come each summer to walk through Southern France. They say, 'We walk in silence, camping in a new place each evening, exploring Dharma, meditating in the beauty and simplicity of Nature, being together as Sangha, a spiritual community making an outer and an inner spiritual journey together'.

In the UK, Buddhafield also run Yatras, often along an ancient pathway such as the Ridgeway. Mindfully walking such routes is a wonderful opportunity to deepen our connection with the land; in some mysterious way it is a bringing together of our 'new' Buddhist practice with our 'old' Pagan heritage: the two traditions need to meet and make fiends and the Yatra can provide a context for this. Each evening, or at any sacred places along the way, there would be meditation and ceremony honouring the 'spirits of the place' and asking for their blessing.

PEACE YATRAS

In the Buddhist East the monks were instructed by the Buddha to walk everywhere; there is not one single story in all the Buddhist scriptures of the Buddha travelling in any other way. In fact they were known as 'Yatrikas' or walkers. This kept them intimately connected with the land and the people around them. Sometimes the Buddha would be content to wander more or less at random, but where need arose he would travel to a specific place and walk there.

This has given rise to the tradition of Peace Yatras, where monks walk mindfully -

in silence and single file - through conflict zones. Walking in such places is a powerful and inspiring demonstration of fearlessness and the possibility of living without conflict or taking sides. It is also a very strong inner practice - the Yatrika will need to be able to contain and transform the strong emotions that will be aroused. In recent times this practice has been exemplified by Maha Gosananda in Cambodia, who annually led up to 500 Cambodian Buddhist monks, nuns and lay people in a peace march or pilgrimage in an effort to restore the hope and spirit of the Cambodian people through territory still littered with landmines from the Khmer Rouge. This has been taken up be Thich Nhat Hahn in Vietnam and Christopher Titmuss in Palestine.

MOUNTAINS WALKING

In the Zen tradition, the simple act of walking can become a vehicle for satori, insight, even Enlightenment. Who is it that's walking? Who does not walk? Contemplation of these and other questions can lead to breakthrough experiences - if you can go beyond the rational mind. To end with some quotations from the Mountains and Waters Sutra by Dogen, a Soto Zen master -

'Mountains and waters right now are the actualisation of the ancient buddha way. Each, abiding in its phenomenal expression, realises completeness. Because mountains and waters have been active since before the Empty Eon, they are alive at this moment.

'Because mountains are high and broad, the way of riding the clouds is always reached in the mountains; the inconceivable power of soaring in the wind comes freely from the mountains. 'Mountains' walking is just like human walking. Accordingly, do not doubt mountains' walking even though it does not look the same as human walking. The buddha ancestors' words point to walking. This is fundamental understanding. You should penetrate these words.

'Because green mountains walk they are permanent. Although they walk more swiftly than the wind, someone in the mountains does not realise it or understand it. 'In the mountains' means the blossoming of the entire world.

'If you doubt mountains walking, you do not know your own walking; it is not that you do not walk, but that you do not know or understand your own walking.

'You should study the green mountains, using numerous worlds as your standards.

You should clearly examine the green mountains' walking and your own walking.

'If walking stops, buddha ancestors do not appear. If walking ends, the buddha-dharma cannot reach the present'.

16. GEOMYTHIC ENERGY

'The human body is the image of a country'. Taoist saying.

After examining the small scale aspect of the physical mechanics of movement we can now consider the environment we move through.

Feng Shui is pronounced fung-shway, and translates as 'Wind-Water'. It is said that 'Qi rides the Wind and scatters, but is retained when encountering Water' (so it is inadvisable to practice Qi Gong in windy conditions, and preferable to be near a pond or lake).

In use around 4000 BC, the goal of Feng Shui is to utilize environmental Qi. It had its origins in astronomy before the invention of the compass, using either circumpolar stars for alignment on a north-south axis or bisecting the angle between the rising and setting sun to find north. In fact the magnetic compass was invented for Feng Shui.

From the Shangshu or Book of Documents, dated to around 2300 BC, the cardinal directions are lined up by the marker stars of the four celestial animal constellations -

East is the Green Dragon, the constellation of Hydrae, and relates to the Spring season.

South, the Red Phoenix, Scorpionis, Summer.

West, the White Tiger, Aquarius, Autumn.

North, the Dark Turtle, Taurus (Pleiades), Winter.

Just as Chinese medicine aims at balancing the body's Yin/Yang polarity, Feng Shui aims at aligning architecture with Yin/Yang force fields, or geomagnetism. Earth acts as a buffer or equilibrium when the polarities cancel each other out. One cause of the Boxer Rebellion was that Westerners were not using Feng Shui principles in their construction of the railroads and other works.

During the Cultural Revolution Feng Shui was deemed a 'social evil'. It is perhaps misused in its modern status as a form of clever interior decorating, and as a science it might be criticised, but the original intention was an aesthetic one.

In Britain during the 1920s, Alfred Watkins noticed an alignment of ancient sites which he believed had been used as points of navigation. He came up with the term 'ley lines' to describe these traders' tracks, to which others later attributed a form of energy (not Watkins' intention at all), so that they resembled the 'lung mai' or dragon lines of Feng Shui. Ley lines refer therefore to site alignment in a straight line, which can include megalithic monuments, churches and natural features. Energy lines are a separate classification, although they can interact with leys. Energy lines can be dowsed and often run through both ancient sites and modern developments.

Dowsing 'taps into' either a form of extrinsic energy or some instinctual sense within the dowser. I had a guided tour of a house on the Cornish coast called Place Manor several years ago where the guide incongruously produced a pendulum and proceeded to locate an area that was apparently a 'hot spot'. There is an old legend of Joseph of Arimathea landing with his nephew in the vicinity; there was of course an ancient trade in tin and other mined material between Cornwall and the Middle East. As far as I can recall, the guide was trying to draw an analogy between the located point and Joseph, wildly speculative as that may be.

It was Dion Fortune in her novel 'The Goat-Foot God' who suggested the idea of lines of energy connecting sites across the country and John Michell in 'The View Over Atlantis' who associated ley lines with Feng Shui.

There are large examples of energy lines, whichever way these may be interpreted, that are not necessarily straight but can curve in places, and that travel for miles across the country, such as the Michael Line (so named because it runs through many churches which are dedicated to St. Michael) which goes from Cornwall to the east of England. This has been referred to as the 'Great Dragon Line', indicating once more a conjunctive ideation operating.

Although they can be dowsed, we still don't know what they are, and archaeologists certainly have no belief generally in them, although they might acknowledge the obvious alignment of sites. Animals seem sensitive to certain areas. They could be a natural feature, underground water currents, earth radiation, or geological fault lines. Even the 'ghosts' of ritual paths that were walked by many in ages past and have their own association of myth, such as the Tinners Way in Cornwall. I naturally have to refer to Cornwall with respect to this chapter as it's my native county, but also because of the great number of sacred sites and circles preserved there still. Some sites are aligned with astronomical events, such as the rising and setting of the sun and moon. Cornwall is known as the 'Granite Kingdom' because of the prevalence of that rock, and granite is especially radioactive, one of its products being radon. It has even been conjectured that stone circles were created as an unconscious means of diverting any negative health effect of radiation.

Natural forms of energy could explain unusual phenomena; another form is electromagnetic energy, the earth itself being a giant magnet whose poles will, as previously noted after approximately every 100,000 years, 'flip'. Magnetic fields are known to have an impact on brainwave activity, and one of its effects could be the humming noise reported at a few sites. For example, when I worked in Cornwall in the mid-'80s I met someone who told me how he'd visited a stone circle at night with some friends when the stones began to make a 'humming sound'. His girlfriend had been with him and placed her hand on one of the stones, becoming decidedly unsettled when it started to vibrate. They were (to coin a suitable phrase) a 'down-to-earth' couple, and had no discernible reason to invent such an odd tale.

These various forms of particular geophysical events and conditions referred to as 'Earth Mysteries' include the appearance of unexplained lights (known as 'Earth Lights' simply enough). Another condition is the 'Will o' the Wisp' that rolls sometimes across moors or over the bonnets of cars driving late across misty terrain, logically explained as ignis fatuus or marsh gas.

The Australian aboriginals had a similar concept of energetic lines in their own landscape with their 'songlines' and, as can be inferred by the sections on Circle Walking and the Yatra, walking along such lines can theoretically activate both earth energy and one's own body energy.

An artist friend of mine with no interest at all in the paranormal was told that her cottage was situated on a ley line, and wondered if it had anything to do with a strange phenomenon she and her husband had observed; when cups were accidentally set swinging on the kitchen crockery-tree, they carried on moving for much longer than was normal. Whether ley line or energy line, this reminds me of the 'token' used by Leonardo DiCaprio's character in the film 'Inception', a little spinning top which when set in motion, indicates, if it doesn't stop, that he is dreaming and in another reality. There have always been tales about 'the veil between the worlds' being thinner at certain locations. Current results with the Large Hadron Collider in Bern are leading physicists to accept that the theory of parallel worlds is at least plausible; the speculation now is upon the actual meeting point of these worlds with our own.

Spiral energy lines are also discovered, as at Chun Quoit and the Merry Maidens stone circle. Spiralling energy within the body is a Nei Gong technique .

My mother's family grew up around, and were custodians of, Gwennap Pit in Cornwall, the unusual amphitheatre where John Wesley preached, and she recounted how, as children, they would run in circles one way around the levels of the pit down to the centre, then race in the opposite direction up to the top. A Dantesque effect can be imagined, to be actually spiralling down into the ground and then back to the 'surface'.

Chinese thought proposes that there is a special relationship between the environment and its inhabitants, a theme identifiable in our culture as 'Sacred Landscape'. Just as the Chinese Emperor was harmonized through a ritual system with his territory, and if the country suffered drought, famine, or other catastrophe he was held responsible, so in Arthurian myth the King's welfare was intimately connected to his realm, and his decline was reflected in the Wasteland.

The Nei Jing Tu or Chart of Inner Luminosity is a diagram representing the mirroring of the external world by the human body, the torso and head being constructed of a landscape of mountains, streams, rivers and forests. The original was in the White Cloud Temple, and the library of the Beijing Chinese Medical Research Institute has another version, with rainbow energy fields. It is an illustration that reminds me of the outline of Great Britain, and the mythos of a presiding genius loci or figure in the landscape is borne similarly by the image of Britannia as the personification of the country.

Ideas of geomythic energy lines can be a way of anthropomorphizing the planet, like the Gaia concept, the lines being correspondent to the individual body meridians. As Hildegard von Bingen said: 'The Earth has a scaffold of trees and stones. A person is formed in the same way. Flesh is the Earth. Bones are trees and stones'.

The association of the landscape in and around Glastonbury with the constellations of the Zodiac, from the work of Katherine Maltwood and Mary Caine, is of a part with the drawing down to earth of the stars in replicated dance patterns as shamanic practice in early Chinese history. Fantasy or not, the effect it has individually is derived from internal logic, just as all fiction has to obey its own sense of internal logic in order to involve the reader. The reader of the landscape enters their own participation mystique.

Anyone can see or make up shapes in the environment which are meaningful; that's how we forge connections with what surrounds us. The objective reality of these matrices may be debatable, but Nature forms patterns, that is quite self-evident.

Another example of the effect of sacred landscape from this town is the Holy Thorn, an iconic landmark on Wearyall Hill that, legend has it, was originally planted by Joseph of Arimathea (he certainly was busy in his time). It could honestly be compared to the Sacred Tree described by Kristofer Schipper in 'The Taoist Body', a tree with strips of red cloth tied around it and incense burnt at its base (an identical homage being paid to the Thorn) that became a village's 'protecting spirit'. This was particularly marked in December 2010 when the Thorn was vandalised. It is perhaps difficult for people outside of the town to appreciate the shock this caused, as the tree was and is a living symbol of Glastonbury's unique identity, transcending religion.

On an exponentially larger scale around that time Japan suffered the terrible earthquake and resultant tsunami that devastated the country. Whether we are living in an era of increasing natural disaster or that the speed of access to global information brings cataclysmic events closer to all of us, our interaction with the natural world seems precariously balanced, a life out of kilter, or to use the Hopi word, Koyaanisqatsi. We can make a correlation between our activities as a species and global environmental conditions, but plate tectonics are obviously an independent activity.

Nevertheless, in broad terms, it is evident that actions have consequences, and human life is not separate from its environs. We are not, indeed, islands entire of ourselves. The value of ley lines and other concepts of landscape energy patterns is, if nothing else, in providing people with another way to connect with the land, modulating consciousness and facilitating communication in schemes of conservation .

17. MAPPING THE MANY WORLDS

There are two metaphysical diagrams which, though originating in entirely different cultures, share practically identical traits and design properties; the Chinese Diagram of the Supreme Ultimate (Tai Chi T'u) and the Hebrew Otz Chaiim or Tree of Life (also spelt Etz Hay-yim).

The Qabalah is a philosophical teaching, originally an oral tradition (the root QBL means 'to receive' or reveal) that has provided a foundation for Western esotericism. The different spellings of the word can be confusing; as a rough guide, Kabbalah is usually taken to indicate the Hebrew religious tradition, Cabalah the Christianized version, and Qabalah the Western magical form. A Kabbalist would not recognize the attribution of the Major Arcana of the Tarot cards to the 22 letters of the Hebrew alphabet which is a correspondence that the Qabalist works with.

The Qabalah used to be a secret teaching. Now it has become a relatively accessible study, even being adopted, in a manner, by the celebrity world as a fad.

The Qabalistic diagram the Tree of Life, which first appeared in 1516, has ten spheres or sephiroth (singular, Sephira) that embody universal and personal qualities and categories of consciousness. The concept could be compared to the Gnostics' Emanationism or even John Wheeler's Many Worlds hypothesis, yet may be said to be even more scientifically elegant, a mathematically precise construct. It acts as a means of organising personal associations into an accessible ordered structure in the way that books are arranged by subject on library shelves, or as the medieval monks constructed their memory palaces.

The primary causative agency is Absolute Nothingness, Ain Soph Aur, the ground of Chaos, from which arises the first Sephira Kether. This is positioned at the top of the Middle Pillar, which is flanked by the positively-charged right-hand pillar and the negative left. The Middle Pillar represents a state of equilibrium between the two poles. Kether is the sphere of creative energy from which arise the other spheres.

Although the spheres can be seen as descending, this is not necessarily a reflection of a gradual decline in the sense of 'The Fall'. The Lightning Flash is the path of descent into matter or sleep, but the Tree also provides the means of ascent as a ladder, Jacob's Ladder or the Ladder of Lights. This way back is known as the Serpent's Path. The evolutionary journey to being awake is therefore expressed by the childhood game of 'Snakes and Ladders'. An advanced initiatory metaphor!

The requirement of balance is represented by the pairs on the right and left pillars. Chockmah is known as Wisdom, and symbolises the archetypal Father. Binah is Understanding, the 'Great Mother', and the symbols for this sphere are the Cave, the Grail and the Sea.

Chesed is named Mercy. It is the building force whose planetary attribution is Jupiter. Geburah is Severity, the corrective which destroys, portrayed as Mars. Too much cake requires the discipline of diet and exercise, but too much of these can in turn cause their own problems. Moderation in all things is the obvious lesson.

Netzach is the realm of the senses and passion, the goddess Venus, and Hod is the intellectual counterpart, Mercury or Hermes. Tiphereth or Beauty embraces Harmony and gods associated with the Sun, while the Moon is in Yesod, Foundation, the world of the psyche and the Collective Unconscious.

There is a hidden Sephira called Daath which acts as a bridge across the Abyss. It is often associated with those uncomfortable experiences and traumas that nevertheless lead to greater insight. The great challenge of Daath is that it is Knowledge, and we have to at some point abandon the rational in order to progress.

The final Sephira is Malkuth, the Kingdom, and the physical world. The Sephiroth are furthermore connected by Paths which have their own attributions of meaning.

An example of how this can be applied in imaginative ways is given by Daniel Banes in 'The Provocative Merchant of Venice'. He makes a reading of Shakespeare's work by giving it a Qabalistic interpretation. Thus, Portia is the mediating Tiphereth influence balanced between Shylock (Geburah) and Antonio (Chesed).

The Tree can be thought of as existing on four planes; Atziluth, Briah, Yetzirah and Assiah, the levels of Emanation, Creation, Formation and Action, the Spiritual, Mental, Emotional and Physical worlds, and relating to other groups of four such as the elements. These include the divisions of Chiah or Life Force, Ruach - Intellect, Neschamah - Intuition, and Nephesh, the 'Animal Soul' which has two aspects, one of which is equivalent to Qi and the other the Astral Body or Tselem.

Another concept of four worlds or 'circles of creation' was attributed to the Druids, consisting of the Cauldron, Annwn, the Abyss or Chaos; Abred, signifying Form; Gwynfed, Heaven; and Ceugant, the Creator.

The Tree is often seen superimposed upon the figure of Adam Kadmon, the macrocosmic identification of the human with the universal. Manley Palmer Hall has commented that the human body is the most profound of all symbols. Information, in the value-free, physicists sense of the word, is conveyed through our physical structure.

Mapping the Many Worlds

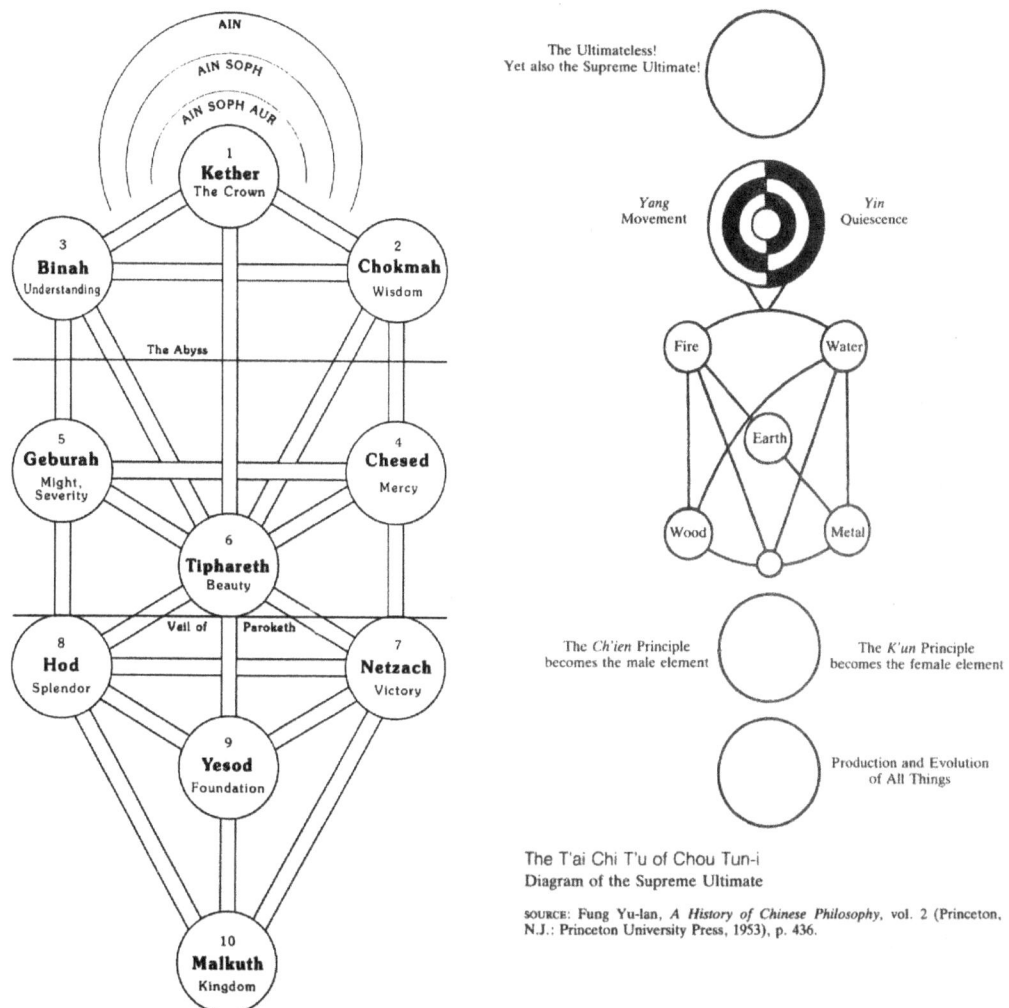

The T'ai Chi T'u of Chou Tun-i
Diagram of the Supreme Ultimate

SOURCE: Fung Yu-lan, *A History of Chinese Philosophy*, vol. 2 (Princeton, N.J.: Princeton University Press, 1953), p. 436.

Energetic analogies can therefore be drawn from the paths and spheres of these maps of consciousness, and the meridian lines or channels and centres of subtle anatomy. For instance, the three pillars of the Otz Chaiim can be compared to the Ida, Pingala and Sushumna channels or nadis of Yoga.

The correlations between the inner work of Taoism and that of the Qabalah are striking; analogous energetic models of subtle lines and centres; the concept of an inherent life force; a sophisticated form of psychological alchemy; symbolic ritualised gestures such as the drawing of a circle around oneself to connect with a sense of the universal; an idealised element system, including the specific Air, Fire and Water formula; and the requirement of balancing the elements, along with the concept of polarity. At the 'high' end, the Qabalah has its Archangels and Taoism the Hsien.

'The Diagram of the Supreme Ultimate' or Tai Chi T'u was designed by Chou Tun-I (1017-1073), a proponent of Neo-Confucianism. The Neo-Confucians developed the ideas of Qi and Yin and Yang. There were various diagrams created by Chinese scholars and philosophers over the ages to represent the 'Supreme Ultimate', or universe, but Chou's is particularly remarkable for its resemblance to the Tree of Life. Or rather, the Tree diagram resembles the earlier construction that is the Tai Chi T'u. Like the Tree it has meditative properties. It should be kept in mind that these constructs are just the scaffolding; every individual has to construct their own building.

The Qabalah was adopted and adapted by the initiates of the Golden Dawn magical order at the beginning of the last century as part of their training programme, and has played a major role in magical and spiritual development ever since. As I have implied, it is in the very nature of such teachings to maintain secrecy for good reason. 'To Know, to Dare, to Will and to Keep Silent' wasn't just a random magical rule.

18. QABALISTIC SILK REELING

With a simultaneous study of both Qabalistic and Taoist philosophies, we find two apparently diverse subjects that have so many points of correspondence, and indeed fit together seamlessly in applications such as alchemical exercises.

Syncretism is not a unique process; during the Tang Dynasty, Confucianism, Taoism and Buddhism were combined to form the Three Doctrines, and also added, for good measure, Ancestor Reverence (the term 'ancestor worship' is misleading, as the ancestors were honoured but not worshipped as deities might be). They all co-existed quite peaceably.

The general ethos of Taoism has always been toward exploring new means of expression, allowing the individual the scope to go with whatever path they might find themselves on and not to shy away from developing and integrating any means which might be of use, even if that development required the application of methodology from other traditions. As the Tao is limitless, so is the way of enlightenment limitless.

The theme of these studies being to uncover 'unity in variety', as both Emerson and Coleridge put it, it's found that the Taoist and Qabalistic paradigms have something to offer each other in terms of an enhancement and greater depth of practice, without disturbing the quality of integrity they possess individually as traditions. In fact the best way to use the Qabalah is by integrating it physically, rather than seeing it purely as an intellectual system and projecting it externally. Obviously, contemporary interpretations and adaptations of ancient teaching are required intermittently to keep up an impetus towards unfolding potential.

Eva Wong mentions briefly ritual movement being designed to induce Qi flow, such as bowing 'opening' the spine, allowing energy to flow from the base to the top of the head, (The Shambhala Guide to Taoism, p.169). This is another area where research

Qi Gong

and experiment can be very beneficial, the overlap between Qi Gong and Western ritual performance. In fact the methods proposed for the development of magical energy, and in preparation for undertaking magical workings, are the same as basic Qi Gong; deep rhythmical breathing and acquiring a state of relaxation.

The equivalent of Qi Gong in the Western Mystical tradition are two classic Qabalistic rituals that use the Tree of Life as a template for energy exercise, the Qabalistic Cross and the Middle Pillar exercise. I will just provide a brief description of these exercises as they are covered in more detail in a number of other books dealing with the Qabalah and magic in general, and that are now available in any major High Street bookstore (there is not a Chinese equivalent in using the whole Tai Chi T'u as a physically related template, but the individual components of the Five Elements and Yin/Yang are applied in Nei Gong exercises).

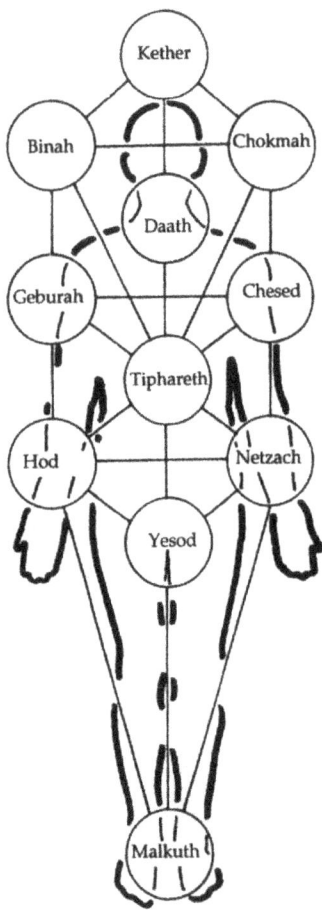

When transcribed onto the human form, the Middle Pillar of the Tree consists of Kether at the Crown, Daath at the throat, Tiphereth at the Solar Plexus, and Yesod at the genital area, with Malkuth at the feet. The Sephiroths Chesed and Geburah are at the left and right shoulders respectively, with Netzach and Hod at the left and right hips.

With both exercises the practitioner stands initially in the basic Wu Chi stance, feet together, hands at the sides, back straight, relaxed, regulating the breathing. The Cross is a variation of the usual genuflection where the head, chest and shoulders are touched with the index and middle fingers. It is used to 'switch on' in preparation for ritual work and consists of imagining a white light being drawn down from the Kether sphere above your head as you touch the Third Eye point. Continue imagining the light going down through the body to your feet and the sphere of Malkuth, touching the navel.

You next touch the right shoulder, then draw light across to touch the left. Finally the hands are brought together in front of the chest in the usual prayer position. As you touch each of the points an invocation is simultaneously intoned, which needn't concern us here. The Taoist equivalents for the terminating points of the cross would be Ch'ien, K'un, Yang and Yin.

The Middle Pillar works with the spheres that relate from the Tree to the human body above the head, at the throat, solar plexus, sacral plexus and feet, also with a set of associated invocatory mantras, visualising the spheres from head to feet. You then imagine energy circulating down the left side and up the right, then down the front of the body and up the back. Finally, energy runs from the feet up through the body emerging at the crown and cascading down over the body like a fountain. This is co-ordinated with the inhalation and exhalation, as in Qi Gong.

A couple of points; Israel Regardie in 'The Art of True Healing' has the energy running down the back and up the front of the body, whereas Alan Richardson in 'An Introduction to the Mystical Qabalah' reverses it. I've used his method as it complies with the Small Circulation of Qi in the Ren and Du Channels.

Secondly, Regardie advises circulating the force within the body, and Richardson describes it as flowing externally, in the aura. Both of these techniques can be used and effects discerned.

Turning back to the Taoist practices, there is a range of Qi Gong exercises known as Chan Si Gong, or Silk Reeling. The name comes from the graceful nature of the movements, the idea of a fine manipulation of energy, as if pulling or reeling a thread of silk.

One set I learnt works with the visualisation or concept of a ball of energy being held and rotated around the front of the torso. I noticed the hand positions corresponded with the map of energy that transcribes the Tree of Life diagram onto the human body, including working on the Central or Thrusting energy channel, the Chong Mai, which translates as the Middle Pillar.

By observing the correspondence we arrive at a 'Qabalistic Qi Gong' which can be of use to students of either, or both, traditions. The subject certainly has scope for further development.

For instance it can be used to picture the Tree within the aura, or Shen body. Alchemically, it provides a means of transmuting associated emotional energy. Whilst in the Taoist form the energy is felt as undifferentiated at each point or position, the Qabalistic model will build the associations of colour, quality and all the other correspondences of the individual Sephiroth.

I haven't modified the core physical movements of the Qi Gong exercise at all. The visualization of the Tree with its paths and spheres can be added as required. The Sephiroth are analogues for aggregates of experience, and are formulated in terms of a range of associations, such as colour, sound, feeling, images and so forth. As example, Netzach, which governs instinctual energy and nature, the world of emotions, can be pictured as coloured a natural shade of green. Chesed you can see as being light blue in colour. The quality of this sphere is expansiveness, wealth, joy. Yesod, gateway to the Astral Plane, psychic energy and imagination, is visualised as silver. Hod, the sphere of the intellect, you can imagine as coloured orange. Here we make decisions, balancing out the instinctive, feeling centre of Netzach.

Geburah, Mars, a deep red, is the sphere of will power, action, martial energy. Kether is the source of your guidance, inspiration, spiritual energy. It is a brilliant white. Daath is the gate to the dimension of Knowledge. Tiphereth, the Solar Energy, a bright golden yellow, confers balance and protection.

THE EXERCISE

We begin appropriately in the 'Standing Like a Tree' or Wu Chi stance. Hands are resting at the sides. Imagine that roots are growing from the soles of your feet, extending deep down into the earth, and that there is an aura around your body. You can imagine this as a coloured light, perhaps golden, white or blue energy. Relax. Take some deep breaths.

Bring your hands into the Holding the Ball position in front of the Dan Tien. Feel energy between the palms. You can 'pulse' this energy, bringing the hands in and out a few times. Now start to rotate the ball, bringing the right palm over the left, then back, then left palm over right. (1, 2, 3, 4)

Holding this hand position, bring them over to the left hip. Breathe down and into it. Rotate the ball, bringing the right hand over the left. (5, 6) Raise the hands so that the right forearm is across the chest, back of the right hand by the left shoulder. (7)

Rotate the ball so that the back of the left hand is now next to the shoulder and the right palm is facing the left one. (8) Breathe into it, and when you are ready, bring the hands back down to the left hip. (9) Rotate the ball, right hand coming over the left, and bring them back to the Dan Tien. (10, 11)

Rotate the hands, first right over left then left over right, and back again. Bring them over to the right hip. Rotate the hands, left over right. (12, 13, 14)

Hands up to the right shoulder, left forearm across the chest. Turn the hands, bring them back down to the right hip, rotate them so the left is over the right, and bring them back to the Dan Tien. (15, 16, 17, 18, 19)

A final turn to their original position, then close the hands over the Dan Tien to store the energy, right hand over left or reversed (see 'Standing' conclusion). (21) Raise the arms out to the sides and up until the hands are over the crown of the head, breathing in as you do so. Again you are now holding a ball of energy. Breathe out as you imagine the top of the head opening up to receive energy. Now breathe normally as you continue the exercise, drawing the energy down in a pillar of light until the hands are positioned in front of the throat. (22, 23, 24)

The hands come down the middle line of the body to the lower Dan Tien. Imagine the pillar of energy continuing down to your feet. (25, 26) Relax the hands so the palms are turned down to the ground, absorbing Yin, Earth, energy and grounding your experience. (27)

This part of the exercise relates to the Middle Pillar, or the 'I' of the magical IAO formula (Isis, Apophis, Osiris), and imbues Stability, Harmony, Knowledge and a connection with Divinity. It is associated in the Taoist use of the exercise with the element Wood, representing Spirit or Void. Wood symbolizes circular energy around a linear axis, just as branches and leaves spread out around a tree.

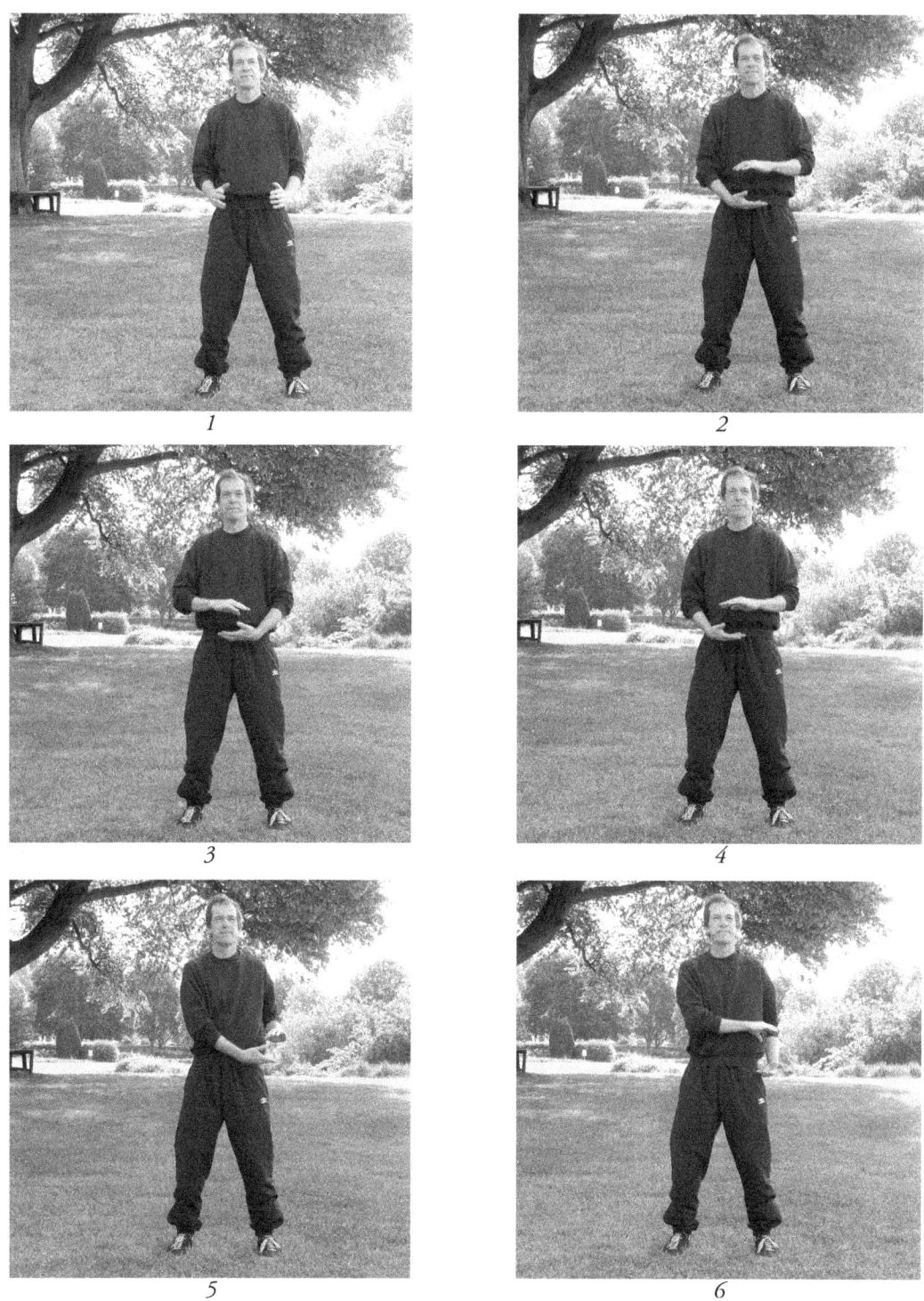

Quabalistic Silk Reeling

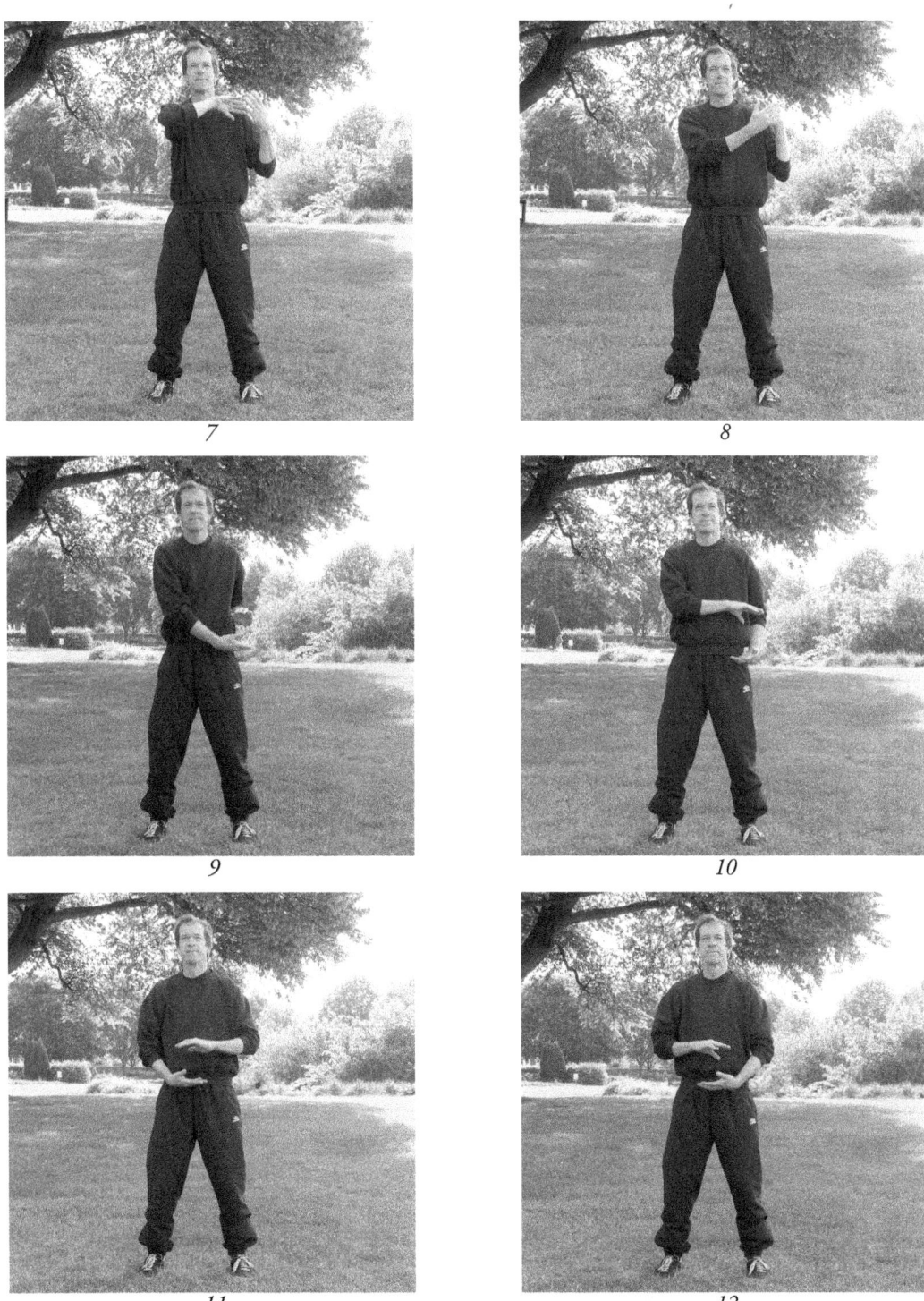

7

8

9

10

11

12

121

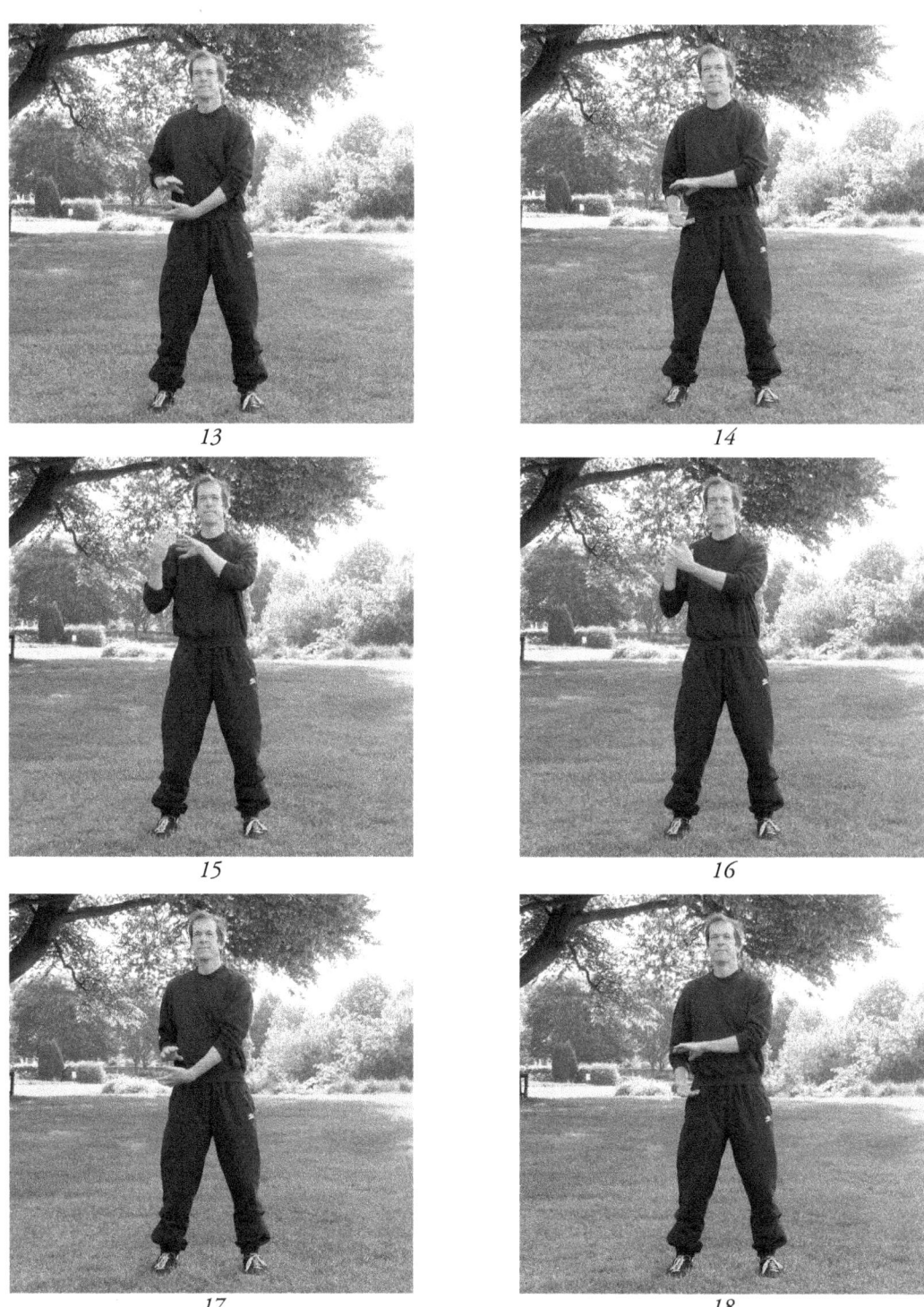

Quabalistic Silk Reeling

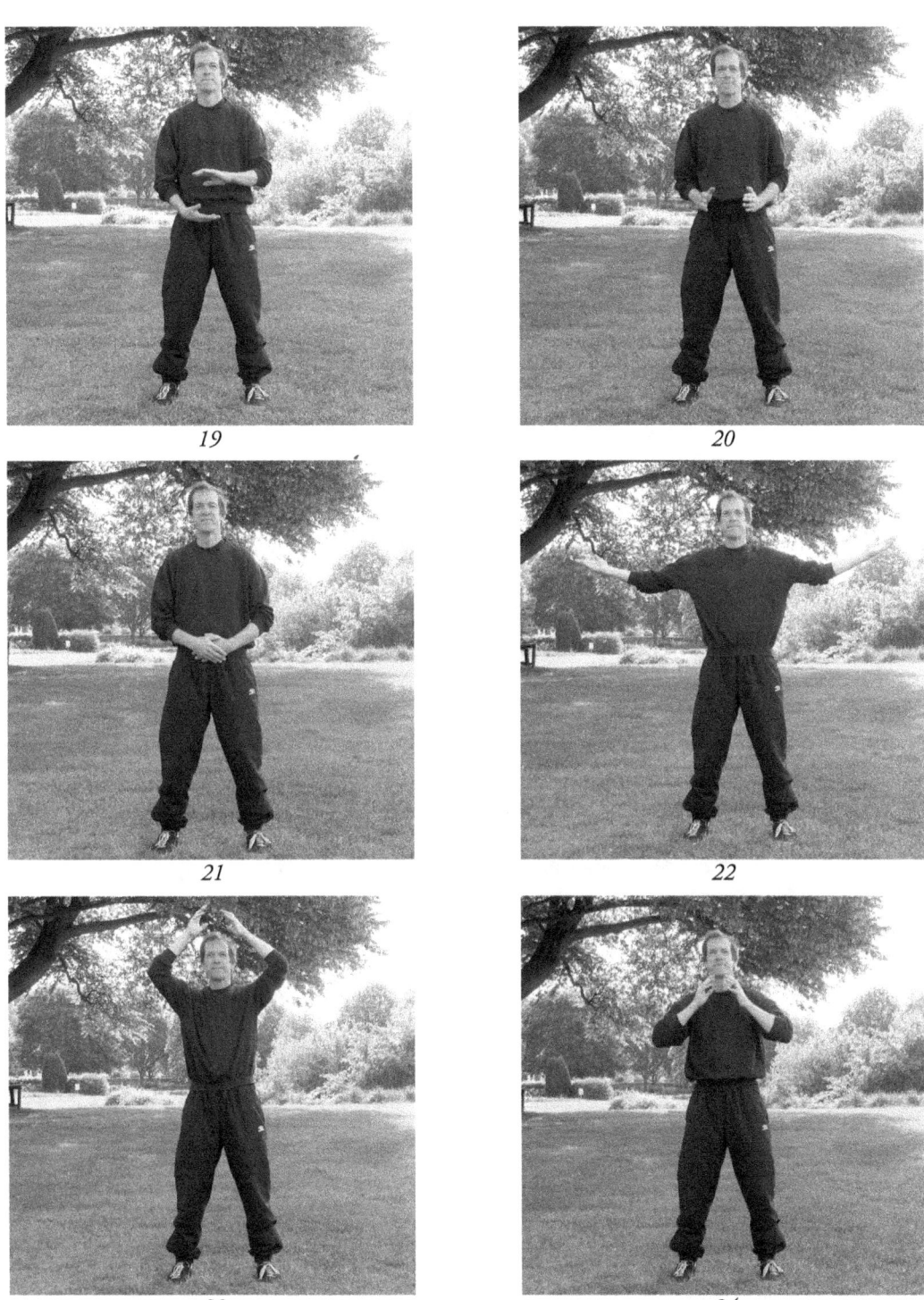

Qi Gong

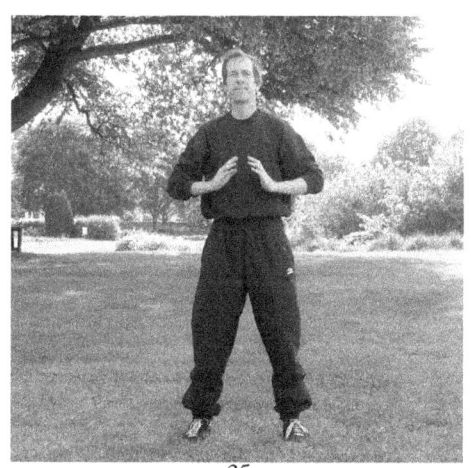
25

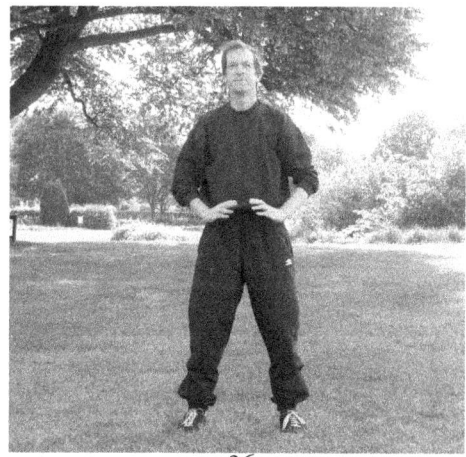
26

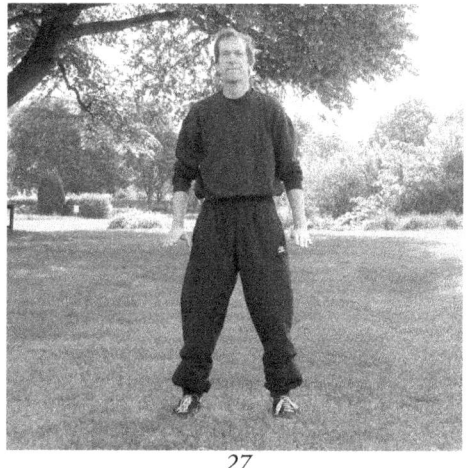
27

19. THE INTERNAL MARTIAL ARTS

'The Scorpion connects with the Serpent through the Dragon'. Dion Fortune.

It's been said that healing and violence use the same energy; it is only the intent that makes a differentiation. Spiritual energetic practices have their shadow side which is just a part of the whole, and a necessary study in order to balance life. The Tree of Life has its own averse aspect. The development of knowledge in medicine and arts of combat became inextricably linked in ancient China; the classic story of the origination of acupuncture is that it was observed how arrow wounds sometimes led to the victim being cured of health problems, according to the point on which he had been hit. Needles were then used to deliberately mimic this effect.

Also, if you look at the Qi Gong exercise 'Cloud Hands' being performed, then look at a boxer punching a speed ball in the gym, you can see they have identical physical mechanics, just different rates of speed and application.

There is even a suggestion, from research by Dr. David Carrier of Utah University, that fighting ability has been an important factor in evolution. By making a study of punching power in different directions he found that a blow from a standing position aimed downward had the optimum effect, implying an impetus toward standing upright in order for humans to best defend themselves or attack others.

As the fighting arts have formed an essential part of Taoist energetic theory development, I will provide a brief overview. It is purely an academic study, and the actual application of any technique mentioned is, naturally, seriously inadvisable. Chinese fighting skills reached such a high level that the masters were often accorded paranormal abilities. 'Lightness' training for example (as seen when David Carradine in the old 'Kung Fu' series walked on a sheet of rice paper without leaving a mark) was exaggerated into the ability to fly, a feature portrayed in Chinese theatre and also quite beautifully by the treetop fight scene in 'Crouching Tiger Hidden Dragon'. One reason for this exaggeration was that the greater a master was acclaimed, the more glory was reflected upon his students.

What are known as the Internal Martial Arts of China are usually classed as the three most well-known styles of Taiji Quan (Tai Chi Chuan), Xing Yi Quan and Baguazhang.

Tai Chi Chuan translates as Supreme Ultimate Fist, and is the 'Mother' art. Xing Yi Quan, Mind/Form or Intention Boxing, is the 'Son' and Baguazhang, eight trigram boxing, the 'Daughter'.

Tai Chi was supposedly created by the mythic Chang San-feng (13th to 14th centuries), a Taoist adept who applied Huang Ti's medical theories and Lao Tzu's philosophy to boxing. It can only with certainty be traced to the Chen family village (there were villages that developed their own styles of martial arts), and from there to Yang Lu-chan, founder of the Yang style.

From him it diversified to the countless variations known today, when it is also known as Loose Boxing and Long River Boxing. It should be explained that Yang Lu-chan's original style included fast movements of 'Fa jing' or explosive energy, and was quite unlike the slow-moving form most people are familiar with. Also it was a fighting art, and the moves were definitely intended for causing harm, whereas the moves now have become shadows of these former intentions. It can be argued that without a proper understanding of those admittedly violent actions, the actual healing energy embodied within the form is lost. Healing and violence are two sides of the same energetic coin, as I previously noted.

'The Form' is a sequence of individual postures that are linked together to create a continuous pattern of movement, a little in the manner of a dance. The internal arts train from the feet up; learning how to stand before you move, and move well before developing techniques. Each posture could be taken out of the form to reveal its martial application and also its healing side. Practitioners were often told by the master to hold a posture as a standing Qi Gong exercise for a particular amount of time, before being instructed in the next link in the form.

At an advanced level the entire form could be performed in the imagination, without physically moving, but the energetic effect would be the same upon the body.

As many Tai Chi masters fled the country during the Cultural Revolution in the 1960's, some of them went to America, and so was created the West Coast Tai Chi fad, just at the time of flower power and tie-dyes. When the Chinese government later wanted to promote its cultural heritage, it was developed as a 24 step standardized or 'Beijing' form. I learnt this sequence from a student of one of China's leading practitioners, Li De Yin.

There is a compactly efficient circular form presented by Mantak Chia in his 'The Inner Structure of Tai Chi' which is most probably closest to the original conception of 13 movements; eight postures and five steps or directions. This is a very suitable style to learn if space is restricted, and it also emphasises spiralling energy.

It could be that the forms became more abstract in order to guard the deadly applications from being stolen from students outside the villages who sneaked a look at their rivals training. Another reason is one of the core aspects of what makes a fighting art 'internal', and that is the training of Instinctive Movement. In what you could class an 'external' art, such as Western boxing, what is trained as a punch is used as a punch. Basically, what you see, you get. In the internal arts, what is trained most specifically is body movement. The reason the learning of set techniques, such as in 'self defence' books, doesn't necessarily work, is because in an emergency situation one relies upon instinct; you do not have the time to engage your mind in thinking, 'This guy is going to throw punch A at me, so I will respond with technique B'. Unless a martial art is instinctual then it won't translate into a fighting art when and if required, and that requirement is often at unexpected times. The Internal Martial Arts are what could be termed 'life' arts, by which I mean they are not studied as a subject separate from your life but are integrated into it. You learn in order to embody the essence of the art. In this way, you do not hold a tense, survivalist attitude towards life, seeing others as potential opponents or summing up situations in terms of potential threat. I've met martial artists and self-defence experts who live like that and, although entirely capable in their abilities, they hold intense stress within themselves. It's not a healthy or happy way to live.

The other two major styles each have their own forms training, but different philosophical backgrounds. Xing Yi is founded on the Five Element Theory and Baguazhang on the manipulation of the energies inherent in the Eight Trigrams. So each style represents a fundamental element of Taoist philosophy (although in a sense Tai Chi contains Bagua in its eight hand forms, and the Five Elements in its footwork). A prodigy who managed to master all three styles was known as a 'Labyrinth Boxer'.

There are particular qualities to each of these arts, and they also apply as qualities of mind. Xing Yi is direct and aggressive, never taking a step back. Tai Chi is deflective, elusive, making use of weight differentiation and the concept of emptiness and fullness.

Bagua is circular and spherical, moving around the opponent and utilising spiralling energy.

In Xing Yi you learn how to punch very hard and very fast through training in simple patterns of movement. This is not just a method in hitting an opponent, but a means of embodying virtues; purity of action and purity of intent. Embodiment or somatic conditioning tends toward expression. Simple repetitive patterns can be a means of enlightenment. There was a monk who only practised one Qi Gong exercise all his life, which apparently was all he needed to reach a state of self-realization. I assume it wasn't just mindless repetition, but an intellectual engagement with the practice, and exhausting all its possibilities and potential. As Thoreau put it: 'Our lives are frittered away by detail. Simplify'. The facility of a single simple movement to hold endless potential is found in other aspects of Taoist arts; the Single Palm Change in Bagua is said to contain 10,000 energies, that number being an expression used for a limitless quantity. Economy equals Efficiency.

We most likely have different reasons in learning the ancient Taoist arts than their founders, for our motivations are probably not based on daily life and death struggle. Some of the masters, to put it bluntly, killed people, and they engaged in vicious no-holds-barred fights to the death. In fact their training methods allegedly included using condemned prisoners from jails to test their killing techniques on.

One of the misconceptions about Tai Chi as a defensive art is that a practitioner can harmlessly deflect an attack through the use of their Qi, disarming the assailant without hurting them (presumably giving them a cup of lavender tea at the same time), and all just through having learnt one of the slow forms. Nice thought, but not a chance.

It seems a paradox, but by moving very slowly one develops the ability to move very quickly, just as standing still strengthens the body, but this strength and speed do not involve the muscular training of athletics.

Partner work, or sparring, was and is practiced through what is known as Tui Shou or 'Push Hands', although that is rather a misnomer, as the pushes really represent strikes. This was developed because, in actual one-to-one fighting training, students were getting seriously injured, so the Push Hands was created as, again, an abstract method of teaching the right way to move.

The Baguazhang equivalent is known as Rou Shou, or 'soft hands', and is performed with both partners walking around a circle. Each style also had its own set of Qi Gong exercises to condition the practitioner. A popular Tai Chi set is the 18 movement form, or Shibashi. Xing Yi's fundamental standing exercise is the San Ti or Trinity posture, and Bagua has of course the circular walking in which the arm positions represent animal forms, that in turn are symbolic of the trigram energies.

Essential energy in both male and female is classified as Yang, so one aim of Taoist practices is to increase the Yang aspect internally. Although I hope the real meaning of Yin and Yang has been sufficiently explained, I will just emphasise here that Yang is not a metaphor for male aggression. The innate capacity for aggressive behaviour that has multiple causes must be sublimated. In ancient cultures, the young men were initially sent to the women to learn how to fight with swords. Yang energy is not the exclusive province of men.

There are specifically martial Qi Gong exercises such as Iron Shirt training which entails 'packing' Qi into the body, and forms which produce 'Vibrating' Qi. Usually these are trained with supplementary external conditioning and are demonstrated by the circus feats of the Shaolin monks. Needless to say there are dangers in such hard training. The external conditioning of the body for combat reasons incurred serious health problems in later years; purposely breaking the knuckles in order to fuse them, turning the hand into a clubbing implement, is really not a good idea. If you get involved in a fight and your hands are obviously conditioned then legally you are placed in an awkward spot, for one thing. Diverse forms of conditioning such as hitting the arms and legs against posts or trees in order to harden them is again not a great idea; a number of people using such methods have ended up with fatal blood clots.

Other styles of internal martial art include Liu He Ba Fa, which translates as Six Harmonies and Eight Methods, and is also known as Water Boxing. A key aspect to this style is achieving a void state of mind whereby the body reacts automatically to threatening circumstances. It places stress upon the intention behind the performance of the form.

Yi Chuan or Intention Fist has a similar focus although it does not have set forms but uses the Standing Post exercise as a core practice to develop whole body strength.

Kun Tao is commonly practiced by the Chinese community in Indonesia and the Philippines, and apart from its combat techniques it has a spiritual training which involves accessing the 'animal' mind to effect a werewolf-like transformation in times of extreme danger.

This last concept leads into the interesting area of the triune brain. As the brain evolved it added layers, so it's said that we have a reptile, wolf and human within us. The oldest part is our survival-instinct driven reptilian brain, which is activated in such classic emergencies as someone being trapped in a car accident, and a passer-by suddenly finding an incredible source of physical strength, ripping open the door. It can be engaged purposely, and the internal arts have postures that teach this.

Russia is of course renowned for its psychic research, and the Russian Special Forces have used methods to access psychic energy, such as staring at one's reflection in a mirror by candlelight in a dark room. After a while a hidden spect of the psyche appears, the face seeming to transform. This could be compared to the ability known as shape-shifting and the basis for some folk stories. The mirror technique is used as a method in magical traditions too.

As to whether it is an actual physical transformation or a change in the internal state of identification is another question. One theory of the Tai Chi form is that it is performed slowly in emulation of hunting prey in the wild, developing a kind of stalking energy that is applied to its fighting method. The postures have names such as Stork Spreads Wings due to the study of animal behaviour, but actually becoming an animal is a step beyond copying them. An example of Shifting into the animalistic defensive mode is the Norse Berserkers, the word coming from Bear-sark or bear shirt, reminiscent of the legendary Chinese chieftain/shaman Yu, who could transform into a bear.

Engaging the reptilian or any deep aspect of the psyche is a dangerous consideration at a conscious level, let alone when it happens spontaneously. There's a terrible story I read some years ago about a man whose wife was assaulted and killed by someone who was subsequently caught and jailed. The husband rushed straight into the police station when he found out they had the culprit, ran past the officers, kicked open the locked iron cell door and, using his bare hands and teeth, literally tore the prisoner's head off. It was later found he'd broken every bone in his leg when he kicked the door down, but was impelled forward by the sheer force of his rage.

The payoff was he actually killed the wrong person. The real assailant had been transferred to another cell. That is the unfortunate lesson of tapping into the animalistic side of the psyche.

Beyond this level is the process of dealing with forms of psychic projection, or what can be considered according to one's inclination, independent beings, and their integration into the self or the petition of their aid. We now begin to move toward the domain of magic. Bob Klein was probably one of the first teachers to make a connection between Tai Chi and Western mysticism with his book 'Movements of Magic' in 1984, but no one seemed to run with the idea at the time.

The projection of the etheric body as a means of causing harm is mythologized in martial art lore as 'The Delayed Death Touch', where a master of the art can project a harmful force, Xie Qi or evil energy, by a mere touch, into the body of his victim causing illness or even death to occur at a set time.

A delayed death attack is possible, but as to it being effected by a simple touch remains outside of the realm of my knowledge, and is likely to do so. The body can be controlled with a simple pressure, even with just one finger, but that is a purely physical application and not psychokinetic.

An understanding of physiological functioning is the basis for methods of attack. The respiratory, circulatory and central nervous systems can be targeted either through a direct assault on an internal organ or by affecting an associated organ using the model of Traditional Chinese Medicine. For example, the brain will recover from a shock to the head by using available energy, blacking out the body in the process, and there are particular points to strike to effect this. This can be one definition of an 'internal' martial art; targeting internal organs.

Some of the points of the meridians that are selected in the art of Dim Mak or death point striking are identified with obvious physiological areas of vulnerability in any case. For example, Stomach 9, which is on the carotid artery. To illustrate that, a few years ago there was a local incident where a man had a disagreement with a youngster which resulted in his being hit on the neck, St.9, by chance. Accidental death occurred a while later.

As to the employment of entities, there are selective methods of negotiating these energies, and whether one believes in their objective existence or not is immaterial (apart from exorcism rituals in religious Taoism there are also treatments in Medical Qi Gong for detaching entities from patients).

To examine how psychic energy can be utilised in its more readily accepted or palatable form as a manifestation of the psyche, I'll give a few examples of somatic conditioning. Because the body has in-built patterns of behaviour, conditioned reflexes, to use the Pavlovian analogy, or somatic patterning, we can manipulate responses. This is a course taken by the advertising industry and other corporate interests in such ploys as subliminal messages. A very basic example is that suddenly holding your hand up in front of someone has a stopping effect, like a red light is also a conditioning to stop.

A projected threat of attack, without even arriving, can have a comparable effect as if it had arrived, because the subconscious mind takes things literally. It doesn't have a sense of either irony or humour, and cannot tell the difference between reality and imagination.

The Russian Systema method uses psychic energy in this way, as pattern disruption, and very impressive it is too when you see someone thrown by a simple wave of the hand. It looks like the person is being thrown by a form of intangible energy, but it's actually a skillful trick and they are, in a manner, throwing themselves. It is a matter of catching the unconscious mind, finding where the point of vulnerability is. The person's own psyche contributes to their vulnerability. A knowledge of bio-mechanics helps as well, most of us being unbalanced (possibly in more ways than one).

When you practice Tai Chi and similar arts for a while you automatically find yourself observing the way people move; weight distribution, alignment, what used to be known as deportment, a lost grace. These are not things we are taught as skills in themselves, and so we go through life stumbling around and taking our ungainly movements for granted, without being conscious of how we move. Walking has been called the controlled act of falling forward, and I must say it's barely controlled at that in a lot of cases.

Therefore with a little understanding you can catch someone's unconscious, finding the point where they are out of balance. Non-physical methods include anything sudden and unexpected, actions or sounds. A shout or scream has a disruptive effect. Shouting is actually a very powerful weapon. The karate exponent's 'Ki-ai' or Spirit Shout is used to increase the effectiveness of an attack, but in itself the shout can cause shock and subsequently physical damage.

An understanding of body language also allows access to the inner state. To demonstrate, applying basic psychological evaluation, artificial movements and tension are a sign of fear. If someone is suddenly scared, breathing stops and there is less blood supply to the brain and heart. Stress to the heart and/or brain makes breathing more difficult and enhances fear, in a feedback loop. So theoretically if you had evaluated an opponent's physical state and discovered, say, a weakness in their breathing, you could use the Chinese medical model of tonify or sedate, applying the tonifying principle by exacerbating their condition.

Rather distasteful as this may be, what I am attempting to illustrate is the extent of our physical boundaries as, after all, without a knowledge of the negative, we can't hope to fulfil the positive. At a certain level all martial arts come to a spiritual realization, that the only opponent is yourself. Realising the interconnection of everything, why would you want to harm anyone else, as such an action is always liable to rebound. Possibly the most effective form of defence against psychic attack is simply refusing to react. This is also a principle of Push Hands, presenting the opponent with an empty space; where there is no resistance, there is nothing for them to attack.

As Sun Tzu stated in the classic, 'The Art of War'; 'To win without fighting is best'.

20. TEACHING AND THERAPY

'Perfect Tao does not declare itself'. Chuang Tzu.

Teaching is a co-operative venture. You consolidate your learning, and modify what you know in relation to the reflective prism of a class. As much as anyone teaches others, we all have something to teach the tutor. It's believed that a good teacher transmits knowledge just by their presence. There is a reciprocal effect, in that students affect the teacher and ideally bring out the best in them.

Facilitation is the essential attitude required by tutors, the engendering of an atmosphere of mutual involvement in the subject. There are no gurus. The Guru/Chela relationship where the student gains a reflected kudos by elevation of the 'master' to an exalted level doesn't help either of them. A notable example occasionally observed in martial art classes is the way some pupils, perhaps unconsciously, 'co-operate' negatively with their Tai Chi or whatever instructor and get propelled metres away by the master's demonstration of 'intrinsic energy' (I mentioned the 'reflected glory' relationship in the previous chapter).

Of course it is one thing to know your subject well, another thing to teach it. Teaching in itself is a skill, and quite a few experts in their own branches of knowledge are not necessarily adept in conveying their learning to others. Subject knowledge is only a part of communicating to others. In modern teaching there are the further issues to accommodate of venue management and health and safety measures (these sometimes reach ridiculous PC levels; when I taught for the local education authority I even had to make safety evaluations of venue car-parks).

The value of the class is, or should be, that the members develop a co-operative spirit, a feeling of support in a mutual venture, and the variety of different perspectives as each person brings their own background of experience to the practice. This is an enrichment of the teaching and learning process that can't be accessed through individual lone effort.

Qi Gong is one of those unique areas where you are not only explaining a subject in theoretical terms but also demonstrating physical capacities. Many students are looking for a health remedy. Qi healing is an unregulated area, so it's best for students to practice the exercises and hopefully improve their own conditions rather than seek a teacher to act as a healer. Therapy is a specialist area; there is, or should be, a differentiation between Qi Gong taught as exercise, and Medical Qi Gong, which is a specific branch requiring as much training as an acupuncturist, if not more. You wouldn't expect a Yoga teacher or Pilates instructor to prescribe for medical conditions. Unless you have a qualification in medicine you shouldn't play at being a diagnostician. Tampering with someone's accepted or unaccepted state of reality is a hazardous undertaking, even if it appears to be an unpleasant reality (like vampires that need an invitation before they can enter a house, you need to have an invite before you intrusively try to heal someone).

As for the attribution of 'karmic' causes of illness popular as 'alternative' diagnoses, that just makes no sense at all and should be dismissed from consideration. If we suffer for past-life transgressions, why wouldn't we be made aware what those transgressions were? Only then would there be a 'lesson' learnt. The kindest thing you can say about the karmic perspective is that it is a misplaced attempt to justify the randomness of nature.

If you are seeking help with a particular health issue from sources complementary to a doctor and choose a Medical Qi Gong practitioner then, due to the lack of licensing and regulation, it is necessary to proceed cautiously, checking qualification and consulting other patients, if possible, that the practitioner has treated in order to guage their effectiveness.

There is also a confusion between Medical and Prescriptive Qi Gong, with the terms being used interchangeably. Prescriptive Qi Gong is the recommendation of certain exercises to individuals with particular health conditions. For example, the exercise 'Flying Pigeon' from the Tai Chi Shibashi set is generally recommended for improving lung conditions.

Healers/health practitioners certainly should not approach the practice from a position of ego. It has to be 'channelled' work, with the practitioner acting as a conduit. There's a divided view on how the actual work is done; Qi Gong masters are not in accord over the source of the energy used. Some say it's universal energy, whatever you envisage that to be, whether God or angels or Heavenly Qi. Others are inclined to believe it's the practitioner's own energy, and they only think they are tapping into a universal source. There is a widespread belief that safeguards must be put up to protect the healer from 'feedback', the draining effect that can happen when communicating with a disordered physical system. What really happens is that the healer makes an empathic link with the patient which can draw out their own emotional states; the way to resolve this is by remaining indifferent. Strange as it may seem, some therapists seem to do their best healing by not caring if the patient gets better or not. This is the means of effective attunement to Tao. You can care enough that you want to help them, but during the treatment session the work comes through emptiness, the inner void.

The technique involved is that the patient is usually seated while the healer sends energy to them through their hands. The positive aspect is that it is less invasive than acupuncture, not even requiring contact. To be clear, no therapy is a cure-all; nature is capricious in any number of ways.

Let's interpret hands-on healing in the most indisputable manner. Qi Gong practitioners' hands tend to be hot (increased circulation). Heat is energy. The patient interprets the heat as healing; their minds are already focused on receiving healing energy, therefore they are effectively creating an internal environment conducive to healing, any positive result being affected through the medium of the practitioner.

In this sense a healer is a projection of the patient, an 'other', much in the way deities are petitioned for help. Many energy modalities work on this interactive basis; the receiver isn't entirely passive. That doesn't mean there's conscious deception involved, more like unconscious collaboration. Most of the healers I have known have been well-meaning people who genuinely believed in their abilities to help others; only occasionally do you come across an egomaniac.

The one time I saw an incidence of positive unsolicited help given was when a Qi Gong master (and I use that term expressly in this case) had 'scanned' a pupil and discovered they had an imbalance in their liver, which as it turned out, when the student went for a check-up, was absolutely correct.

Then again, the master didn't actually do any healing; he just pointed out there was a problem and left the student to seek correction for it from a doctor.

Solving a health problem is not the same as creating health. The optimum approach is in presenting people with methods that may help them without their giving away their own power, abrogating it to someone else. Without a formal choice of health, attempts to improve physical conditions will falter, and the mind can be very resistant to change. That's why we have to approach any attempt at healing or changing any aspect of reality in a subtle manner.

Although things in life can change naturally as a result of structural attention, they rarely change for good if we try too hard to adjust our habits by deliberate alteration. An illustration is the way some people make resolutions, such as at New Year, to visit the gym regularly, or take up a new diet, but then fall back into their former life style. Old habits die hard due to the underlying structure of personal belief, and altering symptoms doesn't affect the root causes.

As noted in the chapter on Qi Gong, in healing one may have to pass through a phase where the disharmony in the body becomes more pronounced, as if the toxins are coming out as a result of the system righting itself. Symptoms can therefore sometimes worsen before they get better. Nel mezzo del cammin di nostra vita, we come across a dark wood.

In some cases an illness can be seen as personified, having its own consciousness, a fragment of the sufferer's. It may be an armouring, using the Reichian term, protecting some deeper level. To conclude, Qi Gong definitely has its positive uses, but we should be wary of extravagant claims made for it.

21. EFFECTS AND GUIDELINES

Anyone with a health problem should naturally consult their doctor before engaging in any system of exercise.

If you are practicing another form of exercise you need to be judicious in how you integrate Qi Gong into your work-out. For example, it can be working at cross-purposes to be engaged in a system involving muscular tension when the root of Qi practice is relaxation. Similarly, Yoga asanas are generally fine to co-ordinate into an exercise programme, although pranayama breath control is an area to approach with caution, and really requires guidance from an instructor.

Qi Gong entails a natural breathing pattern and simply being aware of your respiration. Because it uses 'abdominal' breathing, some students can initially be concerned about straining their muscles or acquiring a 'pot belly'. This is why I prefer the term 'Diaphragmatic breathing', because it focuses the attention on the midline. You don't end up with a big stomach by expanding and contracting the abdomen as you breathe, as it works to tonify the muscles.

Moderation is required as you start, not over-practice. Keep it simple to begin, as it makes it easier to get the mind/body connection and integrate all the elements of structural alignment. Ideally set aside the same time each day as a routine.

Start with the Standing Posture, then add one of the Yuan Qi exercises each day until you know the whole set. These need only be practiced in their entirety once a week to have an effect as they are very potent, but they should be performed in order as a set.

Standing is best practiced every day, but don't beat yourself up if you miss a session. If you really don't feel comfortable with standing practice, then try the moving exercises instead. Qi Gong is flexible enough to allow for the fact that we are not uniformly constituted; there are so many different styles and individual exercises that everyone can find one that suits them personally. Continuous practice is necessary, however.

Little and often is better than seldom and a lot; that is, suddenly being very motivated and practicing enthusiastically, then giving up entirely, won't have much of an effect on your well-being, unlike just one exercise performed regularly. In fact it's as well to learn one exercise effectively than a hundred perfunctorily. Obviously static postures are contraindicated for anyone with circulatory problems.

A problem that is sometimes linked to standing practice is heat rising to the head. Students should ensure they keep the tip of the tongue in contact with the roof of the mouth to complete the Large Circulation of Qi. If feeling energy rising breathe out through the mouth and lower your consciousness to under the feet.

Circle walking is also ideally practiced daily. Some people say that if you practice eight hours a day for ten years you'll get to a reasonable level. Who can spare that amount of time? As long as you practice correctly, and don't overdo it, you'll gain benefit.

One of the most common areas of discomfort is in the legs, as they start to shake due to muscle tiredness and the Qi shifting through tension. Just go with it and try to relax. After a while the shakes stop and you just get a mild buzzing sensation which is not unpleasant.

Qi circulates through the skin, nervous system and bones, and the sensations arising are a tingling feeling and/or warmth, or heaviness. Energy circulation can also instigate feelings of vibration through the body, or trembling. Just observe these feelings, letting them run their course.

Incorrect posture and/or breathing are factors that can cause problems, such as soreness due to tension, or dizziness, which can be attributed to trying too hard to lengthen the breath, or enhanced oxygen intake. As homeostasis is achieved internally there can be spontaneous emotional reactions such as crying or laughing. A natural reaction and nothing to worry about.

At the end of your exercise session it should feel like you've just stepped out of a hot shower or bath. The mind should be calm, aware and fully engaged in the practice. Never try to force energy to move in the body, and breathe fully without forcing the breath. Only breathe to your comfort level; as noted above, breathing beyond your capacity can cause dizziness.

Pain is the body's way of signalling 'Stop'. Discomfort is more like a sign of stuck energy. If you have problems, stop and work out why.

It's not advised that women practice during the menstrual period.

Changes in mental and spiritual well-being manifest in the body, and vice versa. Keeping motivated is one hurdle encountered; as we start to feel better, there's a tendency to let the practice slide. This is the mind's tactic of resistance to change. Making alterations in the exercise programme can help, such as working on a different order or changing the environment you practice in.

22. STRESS

Due to it being such a commonly experienced condition and the adverse effect it has in narrowing access to increased energy I am including this exploration of stress and coping methods. It's not altogether facetious to note that alcohol, tobacco and tranquilizers are one route, but ideally we want to avoid the unpleasant side-effects associated with these.

Advice on stress can seem glib and unsatisfactory when it's made at a distance. When you're in the situation it's entirely different and very difficult to remain objective. Qi Gong can help modify the effects; for instance, because personal outlook on life or a 'world-view' affects energy levels by emotional response, the Qi Gong practitioner tends to avoid restrictive belief systems.

Some authorities argue that all organic disorder and illness originates through stress. It may not be of a conscious kind, but as an example, eating too much of the wrong type of food is placing stress on internal health.

Importantly, it's alright not to be calm all of the time. Alan Watts in 'Tao: The Watercourse Way' explains that the fabled tranquility of sages such as Lao Tzu comes from not being afraid of just simply being oneself. If you are unburdened of the tension of trying to appear to be what you think you should be, then you can relax into the moment.

What is the natural action for that moment is the question, (admittedly, shouting and swearing are at times my preferred methods of coping with unresponsive technology).

It's easy to pontificate on stress and emotions and remaining calm if you are living in a mountain retreat and being fed berries on a gold platter by acolytes. Living in the real world is stressful, and being calm in the face of real problems is a challenge. One aspect of this is the way a problem is perceived. Stress is internal, instigated as it may be by external events. Two people facing the same problem might react entirely differently, and this indicates that you might not have any control over the situation but you do, or can, have control over yourself and how you react.

There is a story of three monks who are walking along a path when they find their way barred by a hedge of thorns. One of them goes the long way around, another rushes straight through, and the third plunges right into the middle, the point being you can either avoid something or fully experience it, even when it's unpleasant and thorny (the story originally described the monks as representing different faiths. The one who plunged into the middle of the thorns was a Taoist. I'll leave it to the reader to identify the other two).

The Taoist concept, or rather observation, of continuous change helps. This moment too will pass. Human instinctual behaviour is notoriously difficult to tame into abeyance. The emotions are like the wild horses that draw Arjuna's chariot in the Bhaghavad Gita. Our primitive reactive drives generate inner stresses that require transmutation for the sake of not only our own health but the well-being of those around us.

There are various degrees of stress and its partner, tension. At a structural level we need a particular kind of tension to ensure we don't simply fall onto the floor like jellies. We can also employ tension in a calculated way to achieve aims, as an archer creates tension in a bow before releasing an arrow.

Muscular tension, increased heart rate and blood pressure, and changes in hormone levels are all consequences of the primitive 'fight or flight' response triggered by stress. Because our bodies are still conditioned for survival actions programmed centuries ago, even though our environment has changed, the activated energy state has nowhere to go in modern conditions. It's hardly appropriate to run away or attack people who cause us grief. Techniques are needed to moderate these innate responses.

At the extreme end of things, we may need to resolve violent energy through a medium other than its literal expression. Venting as a therapy is popular but needs to be used in an appropriate environment, taking care to examine the underlying cause for the emotion.

An excellent way to channel aggressive feeling is through the internal martial art forms. I particularly recommend the Five Element form of Xing Yi, as this also has a balancing effect on the internal organs as a health exercise. Xing Yi being an attack-oriented, 'never take a step back' form of fighting makes it quite suited to channel anger positively and abstractly without employing its devastating combat application upon someone.

If we view emotions as a form of energy it helps to translate them into something less uncomfortable. Detachment can be achieved by using a method from A.R. Orage's book, 'Psychological Exercises and Essays', in which when you find yourself in a situation where you are beginning to feel tense or stressed, you observe your physical reactions rather than the mental processes. A mirror can be useful (and with this you can see how you react by using an imagined scenario, noting shoulder tension, how your face conveys emotion, and so on, just as an actor rehearses).

The very first lesson in Qi Gong and the internal martial arts, and in most complementary therapies, is learning to totally relax. Taking deep breaths in times of stress certainly helps, as you might observe how in tension we tend to breathe higher and in a more shallow manner; our rate of respiration can alter too, becoming faster and irregular. Of course deep breathing can bring out emotion as well as having a calming effect. That is its function as an alchemical, transformative medium.

And indeed Taoist Alchemy is the process of trying to refine the emotions as associated with the internal organs, again through the Five Element theory.

The Taoist Water Exercise simply involves the usual standing position, arms at the sides, and as you breathe in slowly raise the arms in front of you, as if they are being pulled up by strings attached to your wrists. Breathing out, the arms slowly lower back to the sides, palms facing the ground. You can combine this with a mantra such as 'Calm', and/or imagining you are breathing out 'negative' stressful energy and tension, and breathing in calming energy. I believe this exercise works with the Sanjiao or Triple Warmer system, as it covers the lower, middle and upper sections of the body.

Imagery can be combined with deep relaxed breathing in many ways, such as imagining you are surrounded by a protective bubble, or visualise a sacred space such as a wood or beach, or anywhere that makes you feel happy. Perhaps a childhood holiday memory. Another technique is 'pore breathing' where you relax and imagine you are breathing through the pores of your skin.

Using the 'Art of War' approach can be another way. Tactically being prepared, the old Boy Scout motto. Not thinking depressively of the worse that can happen, but perhaps taking time to think of where tension can arise during the day and therefore being ready for it. Of course often we are caught off-guard, so expect the unexpected is another dictum.

For specific stresses you can personify the problem, see it as some embodiment that can then be banished in a ritual, such as by seeing it as a black cloud outside of the Bagua circle which is dispersed by light. To use an artistic metaphor, it's the chiaroscuro effect; light is only made more visible by its contrast with shades of darkness. And that is another reason why stress is so inextricably bound up with the fact of our existence.

Qi Gong

Inescapable as it is, we can only try to modify it and not let it control our lives.

23. CONCLUSION

THE TE: MORALITY IN AN AMORAL UNIVERSE

Tao Te Ching translates literally as Way Virtue Classic. The Te can be understood as the straight line demarcating the Way, not the Sign on the path that warns 'Keep off the grass'.

For it's not exactly the conventional sense of virtue, in the manner of 'doing good', or being bound by a set of commandments. Rather, the natural outcome of being in tune with the right flow of life. Virtue is defined as that which one realizes by following the Tao, integrity as well as morality. Standards of behaviour and core values all stem from the Way.

To the follower of the Tao, questions of ethics and morality are irrelevant, because you arrive at a state where you are not self-involved but involved in the Way, and therefore take all your cues from the underlying ground of the Universal. At this point it becomes quite obvious that harming others has a repercussive effect. You don't follow rules dictating how you should behave, as what does that say other than that you are not responsible enough to be self reliant. Rules and commandments regarding right conduct get broken, because as has been wisely said, 'The word of sin is restriction'.

Self reliance takes the place of the supporting prop of moral guidelines and the inevitable guilt that occurs when not living up to those ideals. Taoist Virtue is not a belief, as beliefs imply their opposite on a subtextual level. Is there anything so dangerous as a 'True Believer'? Belief is static; imagination on the other hand (and I don't mean daydreaming) is dynamic.

Realising and accepting what Robert Fritz has cogently called 'Current Reality' is a means of freeing up energy within oneself, because when we misrepresent the truth to ourselves we are internally bound. The world is not a perfect sphere, neither does it spin perfectly, and by relation to this greater order of things, our intentions are sometimes skewed. Life tends to get in the way of worthy intentions.

What is known as Neo-Taoism, a philosophical trend around the time of the Sui Dynasty, was exemplified by the Chu-lin ch'i-hsien, the Seven Sages of the Bamboo Grove, who gathered to converse, play music and drink. Some critics have maintained that they marked the decline of Taoism, but I disagree. I think their state of intoxication is perfectly in keeping with other traditions of mystical realization, where drunkenness is a metaphor for spiritual depth, such as Sufism. This is how moral strictures can miss the point. The drunken stupor does actually have a profound meaning, as symbolic of the confused state that leads across the Abyss. Rabelais recognized the importance of good 'spirits' in 'Gargantua et Pantagruel', with the exclamation 'Trinc!' En Oino Alethia - In wine lies truth. Furthermore from that masterpiece, the phrase 'Fay ce que voudras' is comparably an expression of the Sage's cultivation of Wu Wei, or spontaneous action. But spontaneity in the sense of that which arises from being connected with one's True or Higher Will. Even, if you want to couch it in such terms, one's Guardian Angel.

The correct ethical code is organically created when you shift to the orientation of being true to yourself, or following your True Will. To 'Do as you Will' is congruent with another Taoist concept, that of hsiang sheng, or 'mutual arising' (the Buddhist doctrine of 'dependent co-origination'), which might also be considered as a reflection of the Quantum Inseparability Principle (QUIP). Quantum Inseparability = QI. Thought and morality can therefore be considered forms of Qi; just as in the Jewish tradition, compassion is especially valued, and considered the highest form of energy.

The gradual decline in a sense of the noumenal, even from some quarters an outright antagonism toward spiritual endeavour in favour of the basely material, has meant that spiritual crises have arisen, schisms that have out-pictured themselves in conflict between churches, pogroms, and the machinery of mass slaughter. An outcome of consciousness being dislocated from feeling and the instinct of compassion. On an individual level it seems there is a constant need for entertainment, as if the mind needs to be kept occupied by trivia, and guarded from the threat of the gaping chasm existing in the heart of our technologically dependent age. The Lottery, 'Reality' TV, sport, are all useful control mechanisms, the gin palaces of our time keeping us safely anaesthetized and distracted. Humanity being eclipsed by technology is a radical consideration, with Humanism being criticized as responsible for most of the planet's current problems, the plundering of natural resources through over-industrialization and the scourge of capitalism. The Enlightenment's Humanist agenda, contriving the domination of nature in order to improve the human condition, was not the entirely negative phase in history that post-modernists consider it to be, if you think of the conditions previous to The Age of Reason. Reassessing humanity in the light of its dependence on machines and the invasiveness of technology is allied with the notion

Conclusion

of breaking away from the dead weight of hierarchical roles and gender dominance. The Inhumanism feared by the philosopher Lyotard is perhaps an understandable reaction to patriarchal injustice and authoritarianism, leading to feminist writer Donna Haraway's conclusion that she 'would rather be a cyborg than a goddess', but it is worth recognizing how the bureaucratic Yang dominated structure of Chinese society sought unconscious modification through the medium of the compassionate Buddha, Avalokitesvara, who evolved through a socially cultivated sex change to become the goddess Kuan Yin, a process of collective psychic homeostasis upon reaching a tipping point. Not exactly the ideal of a post-gender age, but of the genders in balance, or a doctrine of the Mean.

In itself the term 'The Doctrine of the Mean' comes from a verse in the Analects of Confucius; 'The Master said, The virtue embodied in the doctrine of the Mean is of the highest order'. This thought was later expanded upon by the Neo-Confucians to mean the maintenance of harmony within oneself by dwelling upon equilibrium, and was a precept introduced into the educational system.

Aristotle commented on the same principle in the Nicomachean Ethics, stating that Virtue (arete) aims at moderation, or the Golden Mean, as the balance between extremes, and Buddha also taught of the Middle Way. This central way is beyond good and evil.

Gray puts it this way in 'The Tree of Evil':
'Everything begins and ends in Individuality so' (changing the world) 'has to come through individual intentions and directions of inner energy'. As I've observed, W.G. Gray was a magician who worked within the true spirit of the Tao, and so let me end with a final quote from him:
'Blessed be they who are asking NOTHING for all'.

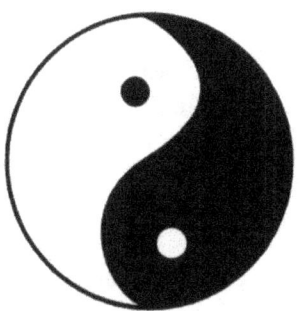

The T'ai Chi Diagram

GLOSSARY

An-mo - Pressure-Stroking, or massage.
Ba Duan Jin - Eight Pieces of Brocade. A classic set of Qi Gong.
Bagua - Eight Trigrams.
Baguazhang - Eight Trigram Boxing.
Chai - Rites of Purification in Ceremonial Taoism.
Chakras - Sanskrit, 'Wheels', originally from the Upanishads, written around the 7th century BC, and subsequently defined through Tantric Shaktism and later popularised by the Theosophical Society.
Chan Si Gong - Silk Reeling, a form of Qi Gong.
Chen-jen - The 'True Human'.
Chiao - Ceremony.
Chuan Chen Chia - The Complete Truth Taoist sect.
Chuan T'ien Tsun - Rotating in Worship of Heaven, a circle walking practice.
Dan Huen Zhang - Single Palm Change.
Dan Tien - Elixir Field. A focus point in energy work.
Dao-yin - Leading or guiding energy. Ancient form of Qi Gong.
Etz Hay-yim - The Qabalistic Tree of Life (also translated as Otz Chaiim).
Fa jing - Explosive energy release in martial applications.
Fa Qi - Emitting energy.
Fang-shih - Magicians.
Gao Shou - Mastery.
Gong - Work, effort, skill.
Hsiang sheng - Mutual arising.
Hun-tun - Personification of Chaos. The Natural State of the world.
Jing - Essence.
Jing-Shen - The Spirit of Vitality.
K'ou Bu - Hook Step or Eight Step.
Lao shi - Teacher.
Li - Strength or Force.
Lien-hsu-ho-Tao - Cultivating the Void to merge with the Tao.
Liu Zi Jue - the six healing sounds, a meditative acoustic Qi Gong.
Lung-mai - Dragon lines.
Lung-men - Dragon Gate.
Ming - Luminosity, or Enlightenment.
Ming Men - The Gate of Life.
Nadis - Indian conception of energy channels equivalent to the Chinese meridians.
Nei Gong - Inner Work.
Nei-Shih/Nei-Kunn - Inner Viewing.
Qabalah - A Western Mystical Tradition.

Glossary

Qi - Energy.
San Bao - Three Treasures. Shen, Jing, and Qi. Residing in the brain, sacrum and thorax.
San Cai - Three Powers. Heaven, Earth, and Human.
Shen - Spirit.
Shen-tung - Spiritual breakthroughs.
Song - Active relaxation.
Taijiquan (also spelt Tai Chi Chuan) - Supreme Ultimate Fist.
Tao - The Way.
Tao jia - Esoteric Taoism.
Tao-shih - Dignitaries of the Tao.
Tao Te Ching - The Classic of the Way and its Virtue.
Te - Virtue.
Ts'o-ch'an - Mind Control.
Wei Qi - Guardian energy.
Wu xing - Five Elements.
Xi Sui Jing - Bone Marrow Cleansing, a form of internal health practice.
Xin - The Emotional Mind.
Yi - Intent. Also, the 'Wisdom Mind'.
Yuan Qi - Primordial or prenatal energy.
Zhan Zhuang - Standing Post.
Zheng Qi - Righteous Qi. Balance of Mind and Body.
Ziran - Or, Tzu-jan. Being oneself, translated as 'Being such of itself'.

PERSONALITIES:

Ba Hsien. The Eight Immortals.
Chang San-feng. c. 13th C. Taoist priest and legendary founder of Tai Chi Chuan.
Chu-lin Ch'i-hsien. The Seven Sages of the Bamboo Grove, who sought harmony with the Tao by drinking wine. My favourite role models.
Chuang Tzu. c. 4th C. BC. Philosopher and author of the work that bears his name.
Confucius. 551 - 479 BC. Social philosopher.
Dong Hai Chuan. 1797-1882. Credited as the founder of Baguazhang.
Hua Tuo. c.145 - c.208. Physician who created the Wuqinxi, Five Animal Exercises or 'Frolics' - tiger, leopard, dragon, snake and crane.
Ko Hung. 283-343. Taoist philosopher and seeker of physical immortality. Author of the Pao-p'u-tzu or 'He who embraces the Unhewn Block'.
Lao Tzu. 6th C. BC. Author of the Tao Te Ching.
Lieh Tzu. Debatable as a personality, but otherwise a classic Taoist book of the 4th C.
Yueh Fei. 1103-1142 AD. Creator of a classic set of exercises, the Eight Pieces of Brocade (Ba Duan Jin), and also possibly Xing Yi (Mind Form Boxing).

A LIST OF THE CHINESE DYNASTIES

These were in reality not so clearly defined as chronologies infer, due to overlaps in either ruling or being overthrown.

Three Sovereigns and the Five Emperors.	Before 2070 BC
Xia Dynasty	2070 - 1600 BC
Shang	1600 -1046 BC
Western Zhou	1046 - 771 BC
Eastern Zhou	770 - 256 BC
(Divided into - Spring and Autumn Period)	722 - 476 BC
(And - Warring States Period)	475 - 221 BC
Qin	221 - 206 BC
Western Han	206 BC - 9AD
Xin	9 - 23
Eastern Han	25 - 220
Three Kingdoms	220 - 265
Western Jin	265 - 317
Eastern Jin	317 - 420
Southern and Northern	420 - 589
Sui	581 - 618
Tang	618 - 907
Five Dynasties and Ten Kingdoms	907- 960
Northern Song	960 - 1127
Southern Song	1127- 1279
Liao	916 - 1125
Jin	1115 - 1234
Yuan	1271 - 1368
Ming	1368 - 1644
Qing	1644 - 1911
Republic of China	1912 - Now (Taiwan)
People's Republic of China	1949 - Now

BIBLIOGRAPHY

Baddeley, Hiram. *Physics and the Human Body*. Author House, 2008.
Banes, Daniel. *The Provocative Merchant of Venice*. Malcolm House, 1975.
Barrie, Donald C. *Bible of the Undead*. Chemung Books, 1971.
Beresford-Cooke, Carola and Albright M.D., Peter. *Acupressure*. Greenwich Editions, 1996.
Black, Jonathan. *The Secret History of the World*. Quercus, 2010.
Blofeld, John. *Taoism: The Road to Immortality*. Shambhala, 2000.
Bohm, David. *Wholeness and the Implicate Order*. Routledge, 2002.
Brecher, Paul. *Secrets of Energy Work*. Dorling Kindersley, 2001.
Brennan, J.H. *Experimental Magic*. Aquarian Press. 1972.
Breslow, Arieh Lev. *Beyond the Closed Door. Chinese Culture and the Creation of Tai Chi Ch'uan*. Almond Blossom Press, 1995.
Caine, Mary. *The Glastonbury Zodiac*. Mary Caine, 1978.
Carroll, Peter. *Liber Null and Psychonaut*. Weiser, 1987.
Chen Yan-feng. *Prenatal Energy Mobilising Qigong*. Guangdong Science and Technology Press, 1992.
Chun-fang Yu. *Kuan-Yin: The Chinese Transformation of Avalokitesvara*. Columbia University Press, 2000.
Cicero, Chic and Sandra Tabatha. *The Essential Golden Dawn*. Llewellyn, 2003.
Cleary, Thomas (Translator). *Immortal Sisters: Secret Teachings of Taoist Women*. North Atlantic Books, 1996.
———. *Practical Taoism*. Shambhala, 1996.
———. *The Book of Balance and Harmony. A Taoist Handbook*. Shambhala, 1996.
———. *Taoist Meditation*. Shambhala, 2000.
———. *The Way of Chuang Tzu*. Burns & Oates, 1995.
———. *Thoughts on the East*. Burns & Oates, 1996.
Cohen, Ken. *The Way of Qigong*. Bantam,1997.
Colegrave, Sukie. *The Spirit of the Valley: Androgyny and Chinese Thought*. Virago, 1979.
Conway, David. *Magic: An Occult Primer*. Cape, 1972.
Crompton, Paul. *Walking Meditation: Pakua - The Martial Art of the I Ching*. Element Books, 1996.
Cooper, J.C. *Taoism: The Way of the Mystic*. Aquarian Press, 1972.
Da Liu. *Tai Chi Chuan and Meditation*. Arkana, 1986.
Dethlefsen, Thorwald and Dalke, Rudiger. *The Healing Power of Illness*. Vega Books, 2004.
Fischer-Schreiber, Ingrid. *The Shambhala Dictionary of Taoism*. Shambhala, 1996.
Fortune, Dion: *Psychic Self-Defence. A Study in Occult Pathology and Criminality*. Aquarian Press, 1986.
———. *The Mystical Qabalah*. Aquarian Press, 1987.
———. *Glastonbury: Avalon of the Heart*. Aquarian Press, 1989.

Frantzis, Bruce Kumar. *Opening the Energy Gates of your Body.* North Atlantic Books, 1993.
———. *The Power of Internal Martial Arts.* North Atlantic Books, 1998.
Fritz, Robert. *Creating.* Fawcett Columbine, 1991.
———. *The Path of Least Resistance.* Fawcett Columbine, 1989.
Gleick, James. *Chaos. Making a New Science.* Cardinal, 1987.
Gnostic Revelation Society. *The Book of Gnostic Revelation.* Finbarr, 1982.
Goodrick-Clarke, Nicholas. *The Western Esoteric Traditions: A Historical Introduction.* OUP USA, 2008.
Gray, William G. *An Outlook on our Inner Western Way.* Weiser, 1980.
———. *Magical Ritual Methods.* Weiser, 1980.
———. *The Tree of Evil.* Helios, 1974.
Hall, Manley P. *The Secret Teachings of All Ages.* Tarcher/Penguin, 2003.
Hammer M.D., Leon. *Dragon Rises, Red Bird Flies. Psychology and Chinese Medicine.* Crucible, 1990.
Hartley, Christine. *The Western Mystery Tradition.* Aquarian Press, 1986.
Hesse, Hermann. *Narziss and Goldmund.* Penguin Modern Classics, 1978.
———. *The Glass Bead Game.* Penguin Modern Classics, 1979.
Hicks, Angela. *The Acupuncture Handbook.* Piatkus, 2005.
Jaynes, Julian. *The Origin of Consciousness in the Breakdown of the Bicameral Mind.* Penguin, 1993.
Johnson, Larry. *Energetic Tai Chi Chuan.* White Elephant Monastery, 1989.
Kamalashila. *Meditation: The Buddhist Way to Tranquillity and Insight.* Windhorse, 1995.
Kaplan, Aryeh. *Sepher Yetzirah.* Weiser, 1982.
King, Francis and Sutherland, Isabel. *The Rebirth of Magic.* Corgi, 1982.
Klein, Bob. *Movements of Magic.* Aquarian, 1984.
Lam Kam Chuen. *The Way of Energy.* Gaia Books, 1991.
Lao Tzu. *Tao Te Ching.* (Interpretation by Ursula K. Le Guin). Shambalah, 1997.
Lionel, Frederic. *The Seduction of the Occult Path.* Turnstone Press, 1983.
Lu K'uan Yu. *Taoist Yoga.* Weiser, 1973.
Lyotard, Jean-Francois. *The Inhuman: Reflections on Time.* Blackwell, 1991.
Masson, Jeffrey. *Against Therapy.* HarperCollins, 1993.
Mercati, Maria. *Step-by-Step Tuina.* Gaia, 1997.
Mercier, Patricia. *The Chakra Bible.* Octopus, 2007.
Minick, Michael. *The Kung Fu Exercise Book.* Corgi, 1975.
Maoshing Ni, Ph.D. *The Yellow Emperor's Classic of Medicine.* Shambhala, 1995.
Neal, Alan. *Ley Lines of the South West.* Bossiney Books, 2004.
Orage, A.R. *On Love and Psychological Exercises.* Samuel Weiser, 1998.
Orr, Leonard. *Physical Immortality. The Science of Everlasting Life.* Celestial Arts, 1982.
Orr, Leonard and Ray, Sondra. *Rebirthing in the New Age.* Celestial Arts, 1977.
Ovason, David. *The Zelator. The Secret Journals of Mark Hedsel.* Arrow, 1999.
Parfitt, Will. *The New Living Qabalah.* Element, 1996.

Bibliography

Pearce, Evelyn. *Anatomy and Physiology for Nurses*. Faber and Faber, 1983.
Rabelais, Francois. *Gargantua and Pantagruel*. Penguin Books, 1955.
Regardie, Israel. *A Garden of Pomegranates*. Llewellyn, 1970.
———. *The Art of True Healing*. New World Library, 1997.
———. *The Eye in the Triangle*. New Falcon Publications, 1982.
Reid, Daniel. *A Complete Guide to Chi-Gung*. Shambhala, 1998.
———. *Guarding the Three Treasures*. Pocket Books, 2003.
Richardson, Alan. *An Introduction to the Mystical Qabalah*. Aquarian Press, 1974.
Riley, Jana. *Tarot Dictionary and Compendium*. Weiser, 1995.
Roberts, Jane. *The Nature of Personal Reality*. Bantam, 1980.
Saint-Pierre, Gaston & Boater, Debbie. *The Metamorphic Technique*. Element, 1982.
Schipper, Kristofer. *The Taoist Body*. University of California Press, 1993.
Silverberg, Robert. *The Book of Skulls*. Gollancz, 1999.
Stormer, Chris. *Reflexology: The Definitive Guide*. Headway, 1995.
Straffon, Cheryl. *Megalithic Mysteries of Cornwall*. Meyn Mavro, 2004.
Svoboda, Robert and Lade, Arnie. *Tao and Dharma. Chinese Medicine and Ayurveda*. Lotus Press, 1995.
Talbot, Michael. *The Holographic Universe*. HarperCollins, 1996.
Tse, Michael. *Qigong for Health and Vitality*. Piatkus, 1995.
Tzu, Sun. *The Art of War*. Shambhala, 1988.
Von Stuckrad, Kocku. *Western Esotericism: A Brief History of Secret Knowledge*. Equinox, 2005.
Walter, Katya. *Tao of Chaos. DNA and the I Ching*. Element, 1996.
Watts, Alan. *Tao: The Watercourse Way*. Arkana, 1992.
Weinman, Ric A. *Your Hands Can Heal*. Aquarian Press, 1988.
Wilhelm, Richard. *The Secret of the Golden Flower*. Arkana, 1984.
———, *I Ching, or Book of Changes*. Arkana, 1989.
Wong, Eva. *The Shambhala Guide to Taoism*. Shambhala, 1997.
Yates, Frances. *The Occult Philosophy in the Elizabethan Age*. Routledge & Kegan Paul, 1979.
Yudelove, Eric Steven. *The Tao and the Tree of Life*. Llewellyn, 1996.

ESSAYS

Cajkanovic, Veselini, 'Magical Sitting'. Translated by Marko Zivkovic, Classics in East European Ethnography Series, *Newsletter of the East European Anthropology Group*, Spring 1996, Vol 14 No. 1.
Crowe, Paul. 'Chaos: A Thematic Continuity between Early Taoism and Taoist Inner Alchemy.' The Camaldolese Institute for East-West Dialogue.
Devereux, Paul. Leys/'Ley Lines': Paper given at the 'Wege des Geistes - Wege der Kraft' (Ways of Spirit - Ways of Power) conference in Germany, 1996.
Fukushima, M., Kataoka,T., Hamada, C., Matsumoto, M. 'Evidence of Qi Gong and its

Biological Effect on the Enhancement of the Phagocytic Activity of Human Polymorphonuclear Leukocytes.' *American Journal of Chinese Medicine*, Winter 2001.

Gardiner, J., Overall, R., and Marc, J. 'The Fractal Nature of the Brain', *NeuroQuantology*, Vol.8, No.2, 2010.

Sawyer, Stephen W. 'The Tao as a Path.' Hanover College Department of History.

Tong, Benjamin R. 'Taoism: A Precursor of Chaos Theory.' American Psychological Association Convention, Washington DC, 1992.

Vandervoort, Larry R. 'Chaos Theory and the Evolution of Consciousness and mind; a Thermodynamic Holographic Resolution to the Mind Body Problem' *New Ideas in Psychology*, Vol. 13 Issue 2, July 1995.

DISCLAIMER

Readers are advised to always consult a physician first before engaging in the exercises described here or in any exercise programme.

www.ingramcontent.com/pod-product-compliance
Lightning Source LLC
Chambersburg PA
CBHW080510110426
42742CB00017B/3056